The Polyamory Handbook

A User's Guide

by

Peter J. Benson

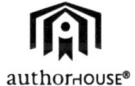

AuthorHouse™
1663 Liberty Drive, Suite 200
Bloomington, IN 47403
www.authorhouse.com
Phone: 1-800-839-8640

© 2008 Peter J. Benson. All rights reserved.

No part of this book may be reproduced, stored in a retrieval system, or transmitted by any means without the written permission of the author.

First published by AuthorHouse 3/24/2008

ISBN: 978-1-4343-7344-1 (sc)

Library of Congress Control Number: 2008902155

Printed in the United States of America
Bloomington, Indiana

This book is printed on acid-free paper.

~ Table of Contents ~

Acknowledgments
Introduction
1 ~ Is Polyamory for You?
    1.01. What is polyamory, and what does it entail?
    1.02. Polyamory and swinging.
    1.03. Polyamory, polygamy, polygyny, and polyandry.
    1.04. How your personality relates to polyamory.
    1.05. Finding suitable partners.
    1.06. Experimenting with polyamory as a couple.
    1.07. Moving from swinging to polyamory.
    1.08. Expressing your initial interest to someone.
    1.09. If a committed person receives an expression of interest.
2 ~ Varieties of Polyamory
    2.01. Many varieties.
    2.02. Polyamory for the single person.
    2.03. Polyamory for couples.
    2.04. Polyamory for triads and larger groups.
    2.05. Clans, tribes, and communities.
    2.06. Line marriages.
    2.07. Intentional communities.
    2.08. The poly/mono mixed relationship.
    2.09. The poly/swinger mixed relationship.
    2.10. Relevance of the term "secondary".
    2.11. From the perspective of the secondary.
    2.12. Sexual alphabet soup.
3 ~ Ethical Considerations
    3.01. Overview.
    3.02. When your potential new lover is in a primary relationship.
    3.03. A "cheater" as intermediary.
    3.04. If your own primary relationship is weak or flawed.
    3.05. Covering for the lies of others.
    3.06. Appeals to protect a partner.
    3.07. Other ethical dilemmas.

3.08. Keeping confidentialities and respecting privacy.
   3.09. Requests for confidentiality.
   3.10. Speaking up with nonpoly people.
4 ~ Sexual Hygiene
   4.01. Overview.
   4.02. Agreement with your primary partner(s).
   4.03. Discuss with potential new sex partners.
   4.04. Genital safe sex practices.
   4.05. Oral safe sex practices.
   4.06. Anal safe sex practices.
   4.07. Dildos, vibrators, and other sex toys.
   4.08. Starting condom use after going condomless for a while.
   4.09. Getting tested.
   4.10. The incubation period.
   4.11. Criteria for fluid-bondedness.
   4.12. Making safe sex more fun.
   4.13. Using condoms among primaries or other fluid-bonded partners.
   4.14. List of STDs.
5 ~ The Relationship Agreement
   5.01. Who needs an explicit relationship agreement?
   5.02. When to develop the agreement.
   5.03. Written or oral?
   5.04. What the relationship agreement should cover.
   5.05. Modifying the relationship agreement.
   5.06. Sample agreement for a dyad.
6 ~ Relationship Skills
   6.01. Communicate, communicate, communicate!
   6.02. Styles of communication.
   6.03. Dating partners for singles.
   6.04. Moratorium early in your dating relationship.
   6.05. Suggesting polyamory to your primary partner.
   6.06. The foundation of communication among primaries.
   6.07. Degrees of communication with primaries—openness and honesty.
   6.08. Primaries sharing about themselves.
   6.09. Sharing about your secondaries with your primaries.
   6.10. Degrees of communication with secondaries.

    6.11. Your children.
    6.12. Keeping balance when more than two share sex (polysexuality).
    6.13. Other skills, traits, and attitudes important in polyamory.
7 ~ Resolving Issues
    7.01. Overview.
    7.02. Qualities to bring to the table.
    7.03. Heal old stuff first.
    7.04. "Hot buttons".
    7.05. Jealousy.
    7.06. If you've "cheated" in a monamorous relationship—preparations.
    7.07. The actual discussion—coming clean about the past.
    7.08. Continuing the discussion—looking to the future.
    7.09. Continuing the discussion—if your partner also confesses to "infidelity".
    7.10. If the "affair" was your partner's in a monamorous relationship.
    7.11. Violations of a polyamorous relationship agreement.
    7.12. Hidden psychological resistance.
    7.13. Moratoriums.
    7.14. Professional counseling or healing help.
    7.15. Polyamory support groups.
    7.16. Growing out of a relationship.
8 ~ Day-to-Day Living
    8.01. Overview.
    8.02. The tyranny of the calendar.
    8.03. The closet and the outside world.
    8.04. In the closet or out, and to whom.
    8.05. Ways to be out of the closet.
    8.06. Your children's schools.
    8.07. Religious affiliation.
    8.08. Children of single parents and in dyadic poly families.
    8.09. Networking.
    8.10. Organizing a local group.
    8.11. Political activism.
    8.12. Giving public presentations.
    8.13. Understanding bigotry and dealing with it.

9 ~ Multi-Adult Families
- 9.01. Overview.
- 9.02. How relating in triads and larger groups differs from dyadic.
- 9.03. Triads.
- 9.04. Quads.
- 9.05. From pentads to intentional communities.
- 9.06. Parental identity and functions.
- 9.07. Living arrangements.
- 9.08. Finances.
- 9.09. Personal space.
- 9.10. Family meetings.
- 9.11. The "hot seat".
- 9.12. Leaving a triad or larger group.

10 ~ Legalities
- 10.01. Overview.
- 10.02. Living wills.
- 10.03. Powers of attorney.
- 10.04. Inheritance.
- 10.05. Owning real estate.
- 10.06. Parents and children.
- 10.07. Hassles and discrimination.
- 10.08. Zoning.
- 10.09. Child custody.
- 10.10. Libel, slander, and defamation of character.
- 10.11. Rights connected to marriage.

Appendix A ~ Resources
- A.01. Overview.
- A.02. Therapists and attorneys.
- A.03. Global, national, and electronic organizations.
- A.04. Regional and local organizations.
- A.05. Books.
- A.06. Sexual hygiene.

Appendix B ~ Glossary

Appendix C ~ Quick Quirk Quotient Questionnaire

Index

~ *Acknowledgments* ~

Certainly I could never have thought of everything that would be worthwhile including in a work of this sort. A number of people—polyamorous lovers, friends, acquaintances, and strangers—each contributed in a small way to this book by telling me their personal stories, reviewing my manuscript and offering suggestions, or recommending resources.

I also want to thank that broader realm of consciousness that goes by various names in its various manifestations—Universal Consciousness, Gaia, Life Energy, the spirit guides, and so on—for nudging me into the feeling that it is time for a work such as this to exist, and for leading me to much of what you see here.

I am specifically grateful to Shannon Hagy at the Howard County Health Department, in Columbia, Maryland, USA, for allowing me to interview her at length so I could get current professional thinking on STDs and sexual hygiene (for Chapter 4). Additional information about STDs came from the City of Baltimore Department of Health and Planned Parenthood of Eugene, Oregon.

I especially thank my primary partner, Deborah, for continually encouraging me as I worked on the draft.

~ Introduction ~

What this book is. This book is designed as a user's manual for polyamory. That is, it is intended primarily to provide guidance for you—
- if you (singly or with spouse or partner(s)) are living your personal life in some variation of the polyamorous lifestyle or in another sexually open lifestyle (for example, swinging);
- or if you are thinking about trying a polyamorous lifestyle; maybe you are discussing the pros and cons with your spouse or partner if you are in a committed couple relationship; or maybe you and your partner have been dating for a while and you are now considering a deeper level of commitment, and the two of you are discussing what your basic operating arrangement or "ground rules" will be (an excellent thing to do!);
- or if you want to have some form of sexually open relationship while your partner does not, or vice versa;
- or if you're just curious about polyamory and other alternative forms of sexually relating.

For counseling professionals and healers. You who are professional psychotherapists, relationship counselors, spiritual healers, or clergy hopefully will also benefit from this work, gaining insights, information, and referrals to other source material useful to you as your clients and parishioners come to you for guidance about issues in their polyamorous lives or in the lives of those close to them.

How polyamory relates to primary relationships. For those who are married or in a comparably committed twosome relationship, polyamory should *enhance* that primary committed relationship. Polyamory should

xi

Introduction

in no way detract from the primary relationship. Thus, polyamory in no way substitutes for the ongoing hard work that both partners in any couple *must* invest in building and maintaining their loving relationship (whether the couple is sexually open or closed, whether they have ongoing issues or not), if that primary relationship is to endure and become richer as the individuals grow and evolve emotionally over the years.

Polyamorists often refer to the core marriage relationship, or comparable committed relationship, as the "primary" relationship (with other emotionally and sexually intimate relationships being "secondary"). The word "primary", of course, means that it comes first in importance; it takes priority over any other relationships. This fundamental theme will recur throughout this book.

Polyamory can take many forms, including some in which all relationships are more or less on an equal footing, so that those involved do not feel it is appropriate to set one relationship as "primary", with the others relegated to a "secondary" ranking. This is a matter of preference for those involved. We will have more to say about the concepts of "primary" and "secondary" in section 2.10.

For any sexual and gender orientation. The dynamics of polyamory are basically the same for heterosexuals, homosexuals, bisexuals, and transgendered persons, so whatever your sexual or gender orientation, and whether you are single or in a male-female, gay, or lesbian partnership, or in a larger polyamorous family or network, the principles and suggestions in this book should be equally valid for you.

From "Square One" to the subtle details. Even if you have only a hazy notion of what polyamory is, this book should be helpful to you by giving you the kind of basic information on which you can base your own choices about how to conduct these important and most personal aspects of your life, so you don't just drift with assumptions that "that's how everyone's always done it" or "I heard someone say that…." You do have more choices now than did earlier generations, and more freedom to choose your own relationship lifestyle that suits you best; and you have more information on which to make sound, ethical choices. And, it's not the government's or your parents' or society's or your clergy's decision to make these most private of choices; it's your own alone, in consultation with your partner(s) if you are in a relationship.

Even if you are not interested in adopting a polyamorous lifestyle for yourself, odds are good that a relative, friend, or acquaintance of yours is polyamorous. Is that person just loose and unprincipled, or is there a solid ethical basis for this way of living and loving? This book will help you answer that question.

But this book does not stop with the simple basics. It aims to provide information and guidance also to those who are solidly practicing polyamory and who (inevitably) sometimes run up against a new puzzle about how best to proceed.

Is polyamory for you? This book does not urge polyamory on anyone. I have tried to remain scrupulously neutral on that question. The general consensus in the polyamory community at large is that polyamory is not for everyone. Polyamorists do not urge society to abandon the kind of dyadic arrangements that have been the norm in our culture, for those who want them. All we ask is the freedom to choose.

So is polyamory a good relationship choice for you? For both of you? Perhaps this book will help you decide, by giving you a candid view of the challenges and complexities that polyamory can present as well as solutions for some of those challenges and a glimpse at the satisfactions, new vistas in life, and personal growth that are available in no other way. Chapter 1 addresses this question in more detail.

I also cannot offer concrete "instructions" about how you can best live your life. No one can. The most I can hope to do is offer food for

Introduction

thought—some ideas for you to consider, singly or with your partner(s), about how best to proceed.

How to read and use this book. As a manual or "user's guide" for polyamory, this book is designed so you can refer to specific segments as the need arises in your life. With this in mind, the book is divided not only into chapters, each covering a broad topic area, but also into numbered sections within each chapter. Each chapter starts with a list of the sections in that chapter, with the title of each section.

In addition to the Table of Contents at the front of the book, you can look up a specific topic or question in the Index in the rear, which will refer you to the relevant section number. The numbering system gives the chapter number, dot, then the section number. For example, "6.09" refers to Chapter 6, the ninth section in that chapter.

Another advantage of using numbered sections is that I can easily refer the reader from the current location in the text to another rather specific location elsewhere in the book, for a related topic, by simply saying something like "see section such-and-such about…."

Some of the sections are fairly long, running to multiple pages. I have intentionally left these long sections intact, not dividing them into several separate, smaller sections, when I feel that the material in the section should be read in its entirety. In other words, whether a particular section is short or long, I suggest that you read at least that entire section before putting the book down.

While this book is new to you, I also recommend that you read through it from beginning to end, as one reads any book, in order to acquaint yourself with what's here. Then later, when some situation or question arises, you may be reminded, "Oh yes, I think there may be something about that in *The Polyamory Handbook*. I think I'll go check it," or "Let's go have a look together."

Introduction

Go through this book together. If you are in a committed couple, and if either or both of you are unfamiliar with open and honest outside sexual activity of any sort, or with polyamory in particular, I suggest that the two of you go through your first reading of this book together. One very "together" way for a couple to look at a book is for one person to read it aloud while the other listens. You can take turns being the reader and listener, or decide that one of you will do most or all of the reading. By reading the book aloud together in this way, the two of you can stop together at any point so you can discuss the point being presented.

Special terms. As for the word "polyamory"—what it means, how to pronounce it, etc.—as well as many other special terms and special definitions, I have included a Glossary (Appendix B), where you'll find definitions and commentary on a number of terms and acronyms that have become commonplace in the polyamory community but may not yet appear in standard dictionaries, or not with these meanings. The Glossary also contains other terms relevant to polyamory.

How this book relates to other relationship counseling books. There are innumerable books available on interpersonal relationships, couple dynamics, and the like. Those books, however, generally do not contemplate sexually and/or emotionally open relationships for groupings larger than a couple, nor do they consider the dynamics and ethics of such open relationships.

Those works are mostly fine as far as they go, within their two-partner purview. For those in a sexually open couple relationship, or living in a group of three or more, the advice given in those books is still generally valid—except when they automatically equate intimacy with a third person as "cheating" or "unfaithfulness", or when they claim that two at a time is the only valid or healthy relationship model.

Introduction

Polyamorous living does not change or eliminate those basic, tried-and-true two-person dynamics and techniques; rather, polyamory adds further aspects and complexities to the interpersonal dynamics that are active between two people. Therefore, if you are living in a polyamorous relationship or contemplating doing so, this book does not alter what you may have learned (or what you need to learn!) about how two people can interrelate well; rather, it builds on that base for those who are emotionally and sexually intimate with more than one partner at a time, or want to be, with honesty, harmony, love, respect, and trust among all involved.

Conversely, if you are having difficulties in your present two-person relationship (or in two-person relationships in general), do not expect that polyamory will let you jump beyond those issues into a new and different form of relating in which everything goes smoothly. If you are experiencing problems in your present two-person relationship, trying to add a third partner is more likely just to make matters worse, not better. See sections 1.01 and 7.03.

Several good books have been published that describe what polyamory is (see Appendix A for information about books and other resources). This book will also hopefully give a good picture of what polyamory is, but it aims to go beyond that, offering thorough, easily referenced guidance on how to deal with the nitty-gritty issues that arise in daily life for the polyamorous person, couple, or family, and insights and solutions that people have found for those issues.

It also cannot be assumed that all professional therapists and counselors have a competent grasp on polyamory and its issues. Many counselors are at a loss when a client or parishioner presents a polyamory-related issue. Many may fall back on considering polyamory to be an aberration, a pathology, to be avoided or "cured" (as homosexuality was considered formerly).

Introduction

I feel strongly that many of the difficulties that people (including myself) have experienced in living life polyamorously result simply from the lack of any roadmap for living life this way. Many of us have been forced to invent many wheels, and, yes, the same wheel has often been reinvented many times. Let's not keep on needlessly inventing those same wheels over and over, separately. Let's become wheelwrights together. I'll show you my wheel if you'll show me yours!

My qualifications. I need to make clear at the outset that I am not a psychotherapist or other psychology or relationship professional; therefore what I offer in this book should in no way be construed as medical or other professional advice. If what you read here seems to make sense to you, it is your decision alone to put it into practice.

My qualifications for writing this book consist primarily of decades of experience living polyamorously—that is, the "college of life" or the "school of hard knocks". As with everyone else, as with all aspects of life, what I feel I have learned in this life has been through partly positive, partly negative experience—some successes, some failures. Some things that I've tried, alone or with partners, turned out not to be the best way to do it. Other things have gone wondrously well for my partners and me. And I'm not through learning yet!

My first marriage was actively open from the beginning. After seven years of marriage, my wife and I and another couple essentially fell in love with each other and moved in together, with our two young children and their three, to form a quad (a four-adult group marriage), and a nine-person family. This was in 1971, when I was 31. Although we chose to go separate ways after about a year, I consider the experience to be positive on balance (speaking for myself, and I feel the same also applies to my three then primary mates), because of the very great personal growth that we all experienced during our time together—growth that resulted directly from what it took to build and maintain

Introduction

an emotionally intimate quad. The kids also really appreciated having four adults to love them, pay attention to them, and help them.

In more recent years I have lived in couple relationships that were polyamorous, with variations on the particulars.

How we all got here. A common myth in our predominantly Judeo-Christian culture in the Western Hemisphere and Europe, and especially in the United States with its puritanical roots, has been that there is only one "traditional" or "standard" way, one valid and healthy and right way, for people to conduct their loving relationships, and that is a pairing of one man and one woman, who are officially joined usually early in adulthood and who are expected to stay together until one of them dies. They are further expected to turn off their biological desires toward others as long as they are both together; or if the forbidden desires should arise anyway, they certainly should not act on them.

Extremists who oppose officially sanctioning other forms of human relating and bonding that vary from that "norm", such as same-gender marriage, speak of "preserving tradition" in attempting to justify their narrow definition of what is the one correct model of a "proper" loving relationship. Yet a longer view of human relationships, both farther back in time and farther around this home planet Earth so as to encompass more cultures, quickly shows that the one-man-one-woman model of relationship is only one of a wide variety of forms that people and societies have accepted and followed successfully in different times and places. Polyamory, polygyny, polyandry, harems, secondary partners and families, intimate groups, homosexual partnerships, nonsexual partnerships—all of these, and others, have been part of the norm here and there, now and then, with various details.

And so polyamory has plenty of history, along with other styles of loving considered "alternative" in our current mainstream culture. Polyamory didn't just pop onto the scene out of nothing a few years ago.

Introduction

What *is* fairly new is the *word* "polyamory", and the rapidly growing awareness of each other among the poly population, and the sense of an identifiable community, even with our many individual variations on how we practice polyamory.

Departing our mainstream norm. A crack in that monolithic myth in western culture about "one right way to relate" appeared in the mid to late 20th century, as many people started erasing the "until death" part, asserting the courage to leave emotionally dead or destructive marriages (yes, sometimes for less well grounded reasons)—though they usually kept the rest of the norm, exchanging one exclusive mate for another, giving rise to the tongue-in-cheek phrase "serial monogamy": having a number of mates, but in series, only one at a time.

Perhaps at least some of those people engaging in "serial monogamy" have been unwitting polyamorists, and that was as close as they knew how to come to polyamory. Perhaps polyamory, as it becomes more widely ensconced as one of the acknowledged options in our society, will reduce the incidence of divorce and "serial monogamy". Therein lies a research study waiting to be done. (I note some other needed research projects in the body of this book.)

Homosexuals and bisexuals pioneering the way. In the last few decades of the 20th century, gays, lesbians, and bisexuals began in large numbers to "come out of the closet" and publicly challenge the requirement that a committed couple must consist of one person of each gender. As of this writing in the early 21st century, their struggle is far from won, but their innate right to the same privileges and legal protections as heterosexuals has gained wide acceptance, and that acceptance continues to take deeper root in mainstream society.

There is a sense among polyamorists that in many ways gays, lesbians, and bisexuals have been on the front lines of the struggle for social acceptance of alternative forms of families and loving relationships

Introduction

in general, thus making things a bit easier for us who pursue multiple relationships openly and honestly. So here's a heart-felt thank-you to the gays, lesbians, and bisexuals in our larger society, who have hacked a path making our polyamorous traverse just a bit easier!

Challenging the twosome monopoly. As gays, lesbians, and bisexuals have become far more ready to come out of the closet and struggle against bigoted restrictions against them, another emerging social phenomenon in the second half of the 20th century was initially called "open marriage" or "open relationships"—the idea that spouses (or committed unmarried partners) could agree to be free to share sex with others, openly and honestly, that is, without the lying and secrecy and blame and guilt that traditionally accompany "affairs" under the mainstream norm that decrees that spouses or committed partners must always be sexually exclusive with each other, so that any departure from that norm must be kept secret from one's partner and everyone else. (See section 1.01.)

The practice of sexually open relationships of whatever sort, not surprisingly, was met with resistance of the same sort that gays, lesbians, and bisexuals faced, from those who would prefer that everyone be stamped from the same cookie cutter—the cookie cutter from which *they* were stamped, of course. Thus, those who have practiced sexually open relationships of any variety, or wanted to, have faced many of the same obstacles and issues in society at large that gays, lesbians, and bisexuals have faced since even earlier.

But the struggle still is far from over, both for gays, lesbians, and bisexuals and for those in open relationships.

The bigger picture. In Chapter 6, talking about human interconnections in twosomes and larger groups, I use a metaphor from chemistry, referring to individuals as "atoms" and couples and larger committed groups as "molecules". This metaphor is actually quite close.

Introduction

In any chemical molecule (containing two atoms, three, or thousands), each atom exchanges energy with the others in such a way as to create the chemical bonds that hold the atoms together in the molecule. These energy connections are actually called "bonds" in chemistry—a perfectly good term also among human beings.

Again with people as with atoms, more and more complex bondings are possible with larger and larger numbers; and along with the bondings come ever more complex and sophisticated interactions and capabilities. Think of a bag containing thousands of loose atoms of carbon, oxygen, nitrogen, etc., and what each atom can do separately—not much. Think of those atoms joined together in the particular pattern that we call a molecule of deoxyribonucleic acid (DNA). Now these same atoms together can contain every possible variation of genetic information. Think of many DNA molecules of different types forming a human body. Now this very special and specialized collection of atoms has enough complexity that it can serve as host for a conscious entity, a human mind and spirit.

Our dominant western culture for a number of centuries has repressed the formation of human "molecules" larger than two "atoms"—the equivalent of carbon monoxide or table salt. Now many people are rejecting those limitations and exploring the possibilities of combining three people, or four, or more. What are we in the process of evolving here? We cannot know, any more than a molecule of water (three atoms) or methane (five) can anticipate a DNA molecule or a human body or human mind.

But something big is stirring—and we're all part of it.

Where we're headed. Some segments of society, enslaved by their own unconscious fears, would impose a repressive theocracy with its attendant tight restrictions on people's rights and lifestyle choices—but it seems inevitable that the future (maybe in stops and starts) will see

Introduction

a continuation of the great blossoming that we're already seeing in the varieties of ways in which people choose to live together and love together. The seeds have sprouted, the land is turning green everywhere we look, and nothing can stop that.

As people experiment, as with all experiments, some emotional paths will lead to greater fulfillment, love, and growth, and some will be dead-ends. A fulfilling, growthful path for one may be a dead-end for another, and vice versa. The goal of this book is to serve as a guide for you, the pioneers along those new paths.

Distinguishing polyamory from swinging. Gradually, roughly during the last two decades of the 20th century, many people in "open relationships" began to distinguish whether their outside sexual involvements were based primarily on the enjoyment of sex with a variety of partners, with lesser importance for any emotional connectedness of the partners; or on caring, loving bonds developed openly and honestly with more than one partner at a time. The sex-focused open relationships came to be known as "swinging" (a vast improvement over the horrendously sexist earlier term, "wife-swapping", dating from the 1940s or 1950s).

The term "polyamory" first appeared publicly in 1990 to describe open relationships in which the primary importance lay with *emotional* connectedness, but in which multiple sexual involvement was also accepted, when done openly and honestly. (See the Glossary entry for *polyamory*.)

There is more discussion comparing swinging with polyamory in section 1.02.

Your input is invited. The book you now hold is the first edition of this handbook. Hopefully it will not be the last. Although I have had wonderful contributions and suggestions from a number of polyamorous people and others in preparing this guide, it would still be impossible, obviously, to think of everything. You may also have different ideas

Introduction

about how to handle a given situation that I do treat here. You may want to let readers know about a book, organization, website, etc., that I did not mention in the appendices.

For these reasons I eagerly encourage you to give me feedback about how this book could be improved for future editions. You can contact me by writing to me at petebenson@starpower.net. In the event that address proves to be not valid at some time in the future, I suggest that you try contacting the publisher, AuthorHouse (www.authorhouse.com, 888-519-5121 in the U.S.), for updated contact information for me (or perhaps for someone else who may take over responsibility for future revisions), or send your comments to the publisher for forwarding to me or the appropriate person.

May you always find more love!

Pete Benson

~ 1 ~
Is Polyamory for You?

Contents:
1.01. What is polyamory, and what does it entail?
1.02. Polyamory and swinging.
1.03. Polyamory, polygamy, polygyny, and polyandry.
1.04. How your personality relates to polyamory.
1.05. Finding suitable partners.
1.06. Experimenting with polyamory as a couple.
1.07. Moving from swinging to polyamory.
1.08. Expressing your initial interest to someone.
1.09. If a committed person receives an expression of interest.

1.01. What is polyamory, and what does it entail?

Polyamory is not a "license for affairs". The term "polyamory" (from Greek and Latin roots meaning "many loves") means the practice or theory of having emotionally intimate relationships with more than one person simultaneously, with sex as a permissible expression of the caring feelings, openly and honestly keeping one's primary partner or partners (or dating partners) informed of the existence of other intimate involvements. See the entry for "polyamory" in the Glossary (Appendix B) for further discussion of the term, its history, etc.

Having two or more simultaneous *relationships* that include sex does not necessarily mean sharing sex with all of one's *partners* simultaneously,

1.01

although that's one option if desired. See Chapter 2 for more about the varieties of polyamory.

Polyamorous relationships may be emotional without sex, but it is understood that sexual expression is at least an accepted option, with conditions and limits agreed by all parties concerned. Polyamory is egalitarian between the genders (not sexist).

"What's new about outside relationships?" you may well ask; "People have been doing that since time immemorial."

Quite true, and that fact—in the face of taboos in many cultures against it—shows just how strongly innate is the human urge toward loving other people and sharing sex with other people, not limited to just one partner. But the phrases "emotionally intimate" and "openly and honestly" in the definition above make all the difference. So, polyamory is *not* about indiscriminate sex with many partners, and it is *not* about secret affairs.

Consequences of lying. In contrast to the expectation of "openness and honesty" in polyamory, the term "affair" usually implies lying and secrecy by one partner in a couple toward the other. When the other partner learns of the affair, they (meaning "he or she" in this singular sense) naturally feel hurt and betrayed; their trust in their partner is seriously stressed at best, and may be irrevocably shattered. Meanwhile, the transgressor probably feels guilt to some degree for having violated the commitment vow or promise to be sexually exclusive. It is known in psychology that negative feelings about oneself, such as guilt or self-criticism, often unconsciously lead that person to feel and behave badly toward the mistreated party—their spouse or partner in this case—projecting the uncomfortable negative feelings about oneself outward onto someone else, ascribing those feelings instead to the other person.

Even if the mistreated partner never explicitly learns of the other partner's affair, the transgressor's bad feelings and behavior resulting from guilt and self-criticism are likely to be manifested, at least indirectly, causing disruption and strife and thus undermining the relationship. (But be careful: There certainly are many other causes of relationship strife. If your partner seems to be picking arguments with you, that in no way means that he or she is having a secret affair!)

It is no surprise, then, that secret sexual affairs lead to the break-up of many basically good and sound relationships. After an affair, the primary relationship often can be salvaged only through serious hard work and much good will by both partners—by the transgressor to rebuild trustworthiness and relieve their own guilt and self-esteem, by the aggrieved to come to feel that they can trust their partner again, and maybe rebuild their own self-esteem as well.

Polyamory does not condone additional relationships based on this sort of secrecy, lying, and betrayal of trust. It does not say, "Follow your whim of the moment, and damn the consequences." Rather, polyamory takes a closer look at what is really the culprit in these situations.

What's behind the betrayal. It's important to realize at the outset what does and does not underlie this betrayal and sense of shattered trust. The culprit is not the outside sexual involvement or loving feelings for someone else. That does not go deep enough. The culprit is the lying and secrecy, and the fact of having violated an agreement or vow, which leads directly to the feelings of guilt by one partner and betrayal by the other, and all the rest, like a chain of dominos.

The way out. Polyamory addresses the problem at its true core, the lying and secrecy, and the content of the vow or agreement. It does so not by puritanically urging stricter behavior, saying that one should scrupulously resist temptation and restrict oneself to one emotional and sexual partner—which just generates frustration and usually does not

1.01

work anyway, since it appears to contravene a basic aspect of human nature. Rather, polyamory affirms the ethical need for openness and honesty, allowing partners to give each other more options for the relationship agreement, right along with the multiple relationships. (See Chapter 3 for more about ethical considerations.)

To be sure, openness and honesty alone are not enough to live polyamorously with joy and love. (If it were, this manual would be a pamphlet ending here, not a book-length guide!) But openness and honesty are twin cornerstones. Never lie to your partner. Never withhold information or tell half-truths that would lead your partner to come to erroneous conclusions. Such withholding of information is tantamount to lying, and lying in any form is deeply destructive of your primary relationship.

These twin concepts of openness and honesty are dealt with more completely in section 6.07.

Keep maintaining your primary relationship. We cannot leave this topic without mentioning another cornerstone that is at least as important as openness and honesty. That is the need to continuously work on and strengthen your marriage or your primary relationship (if you are in such a relationship), continuously reassuring your primary partner (or partners, if you are in a triad etc.)—in a sincere, believable way—that he or she or they are central to your own life, the one(s) most important to you. Of course this is also very important in monamorous (sexually exclusive) relationships, but it becomes even more important when additional loving relationships enter the picture.

When your relationship runs into bumps in the road, work diligently together with your partner(s) to overcome the problems. Get professional counseling if you have difficulty resolving problems on your own. Don't just let things ride or ignore them. Some local polyamory groups also provide "support groups" in which you can share your problems confidentially and get sympathetic and constructive suggestions—or empathy at the least! See Appendix A for more about resources.

This book also goes into more detail about how to do that maintenance work. In a sense, this entire book (the same as many other books of relationship advice) is about building and maintaining your *primary* relationship. In this book, Chapter 6 is focused most specifically on building and using relationship skills.

Degrees of complexity. The complexity of relationships goes up exponentially as more people become involved. In a couple, there is only one relationship, the one between the two people involved. In a triad, with only one additional person, the number of relationships jumps to *four:* there are three twosome relationships (between A-B, A-C, and B-C) and the threesome relationship. (A "relationship" exists between any two primary partners whether they share sex with each other or not.) In a quad, larger by one more person, there are six twosome relationships, four threesomes, plus the foursome, for a total of *eleven* relationships, all in the one quad! And that counts only the *primary* relationships, before you start thinking about adding secondary relationships.

You can amuse yourself by calculating the number of primary relationships in larger committed groupings, five on up, using a calculator and a sketchpad.

Not just the number of relationships increases as more members are added to the partnership, but new *kinds* of interactions come into play. These are discussed in more detail in section 9.02 and elsewhere in Chapter 9.

Physical variations and limitations. Polyamorists have likes, dislikes, and preferences as much as anyone else regarding the bodily characteristics of those they become intimate with, but because polyamory emphasizes emotional connectedness, relatively less importance is usually given to

5

physical characteristics. Polyamorists span the same spectrum as the population as a whole in terms of age, body type and fitness, weight, physical limitations, ethnic ancestry, etc. We have the same paunches, baldness, sagging breasts, wrinkles, surgical scars, amputations, wheelchairs and prostheses—or smooth skin, tight abs, perky tits, luxuriant hair, sleek build, strength and stamina. You will be welcomed into your local poly group for the person that you are, regardless of your physical appearance or any limitations.

Polyamory can be hard work. You can see from the above that, while polyamory does promise greatly widened personal horizons, satisfactions, personal growth, and lots of just plain fun, it can also come with a price—lots of emotional work, for yourself and your partner(s). How much work? That can vary widely. Some people seem to breeze along relatively easily, although even for them there is effort required, for discussing details and variations with partners, for scheduling multiple relationships on the calendar, etc. Others need to apply a *lot* of personal work, involving considerable personal growth and change. Of course this is a very worthy endeavor in its own right, as well as being very satisfying.

So, as you address the question, "Is polyamory for me?" consider whether you are willing to put in the effort required as well as whether you are temperamentally suited for it (discussed below in section 1.03).

1.02.   Polyamory and swinging.

How are polyamory and swinging similar, and how do they differ? Polyamory and swinging have similarities and differences. In the discussion that follows, keep in mind that comparisons between polyamory and swinging can only be general and approximate at best. Everyone has their own preferred style of relating. Like other spectra of relating, such as homosexuality/heterosexuality or sexual exclusivity or multiplicity, everyone who pursues multiple relationships falls somewhere along a spectrum between pure polyamory and pure swinging (whatever "purity" might mean here). Some who identify themselves as "swingers" follow a personal practice that would look like polyamory to others, and vice versa for some who call themselves "polyamorists".

The primary similarity is that both polyamory and swinging affirm that committed partners can enjoy multiple sexual involvements, provided that everyone is open and honest and in agreement about their activities, without threatening to destroy the primary relationship—perhaps strengthening and enriching it.

Another similarity is that both swingers and polyamorists span the entire adult age range in good numbers.

The differences are a matter of emphasis more than of fundamental philosophy. Some of these differences are rather basic; some are more subtle. Some confirmed polyamorists would never dream of attending a swingers' sex party or engaging in a one-night stand on a whim; some confirmed swingers have no interest in developing multiple ongoing caring relationships.

The most fundamental difference (something of an oversimplification) is that polyamory emphasizes caring emotional connectedness with multiple partners; swinging emphasizes sex with a variety of partners for its own intrinsic enjoyment. In polyamory, sex then becomes an accepted expression of the caring relationships that have arisen—or sex sometimes does not happen at all; a strong caring friendship can arise and continue without sexual expression. In swinging, sex may sometimes be added to an existing friendship, but typically the sexual connection comes first or may come after only superficially getting acquainted, and then a friendship or stronger feelings may arise with someone later, after repeated sexual encounters—or may never develop beyond a rather superficial acquaintanceship. One-night stands, casual connections at a party, etc., are common in swinging, more rare in polyamory.

As mentioned, there are other differences of a more indirect or subtle nature. Much of what follows here is just a matter of my subjective impressions. (These questions would make an excellent academic research study in sociology, or series of studies.)

Swinging tends to be a phenomenon done by and among couples, with occasional singles joining a couple for momentary threesome fun, especially single women, since far more swinging couples seem to seek sexual threesomes by adding another woman than by adding a man. Swinging organizations or clubs often have explicit barriers against single men participating except in small numbers. One almost never hears of primary (cohabiting, committed) triads or larger primary groups in swinging. Swinging couples generally "play" together, with another couple or with a single; they do not often have dates involving only one member of the couple plus a third person.

In polyamory, couples may also be the most common combination, but single men as well as women are common, as are triads and quads. Larger cohabiting and sexually involved groups and networks are often seen in polyamory communities. Single men are not shunned in polyamory. Gays and lesbians are also common and welcomed in poly groups.

The reason for the different treatment of single men among swingers and polyamorists may be (author's conjecture) the perception that single men seek quick sexual connections more commonly than do single women, less commonly are interested in the longer-term effort of developing emotional connectedness with someone else. This may lead a group of swingers, where quick sex is more the norm, to perceive that there are too many single men compared with single women interested in joining them, so that the single men come to be seen as an annoyance and are not welcomed.

Some other differences between polyamory and swinging are even more in the realm of the author's impression or conjecture (yet more room for future research studies). Swingers (author's impression) seem to be more often political and religious conservatives, traditional or mainstream in their lifestyles in ways other than sexual. Swingers are more often Christians and Republicans (in the U.S.) or Conservatives (Canada etc.). Polyamorists tend to be more progressive and experimentational not just in their sexual relationships but also in politics and religion, and in life in general. In their spiritual practices, polyamorists are often Pagans, Unitarian-Universalists, Reform Jews, Buddhists, atheists, or "spiritual but not religious". Politically they are more often Democrats (in the U.S.), Liberals, or otherwise left of center.

1.03. Polyamory, polygamy, polygyny, and polyandry.

Some people confuse polyamory with polygamy, and confuse polygamy in turn with polygyny.

"Polygamy" means having more than one legally registered spouse at a time. In most or all western cultures, this is illegal. Polygamy encompasses both polygyny (a man having more than one wife at a time) and polyandry (a woman having more than one husband), but many people in our culture, when they hear the term "polygamy", automatically think only of a man having multiple wives, not considering the possibility of a woman having multiple husbands.

This confusion is probably rooted in the pervasive male-centric sexism in our culture. It may have been exacerbated by the practice of polygamy by some Mormons (Church of Latter Day Saints, LDS) in the 19th century (with pockets of the practice continuing to this day). Among Mormons, polygamy always involved one man with multiple wives (strictly speaking, polygyny); a woman in the Church of LDS was never allowed to have multiple husbands (polyandry).

Polyamory, on the other hand, is gender-egalitarian, as noted in the definition in section 1.01. Women are about as numerous as men in the overall polyamory community, and show as much desire as men to take on multiple romantic and sexual relationships.

Polyamory is also not involved with *legal* status—as to whether one's loving partners are married to each other as husbands or wives. Polyamory has to do with *emotional and sexual partnerships,* regardless of whether a partnership is sanctioned by a religious institution and/or registered with the government as a marriage.

1.04. How your personality relates to polyamory.

Not for everyone. The basic description of polyamory in section 1.01 may sound good in theory (intellectually), but people with the best of intentions sometimes give polyamory a try, or just contemplate it, and they find that their gut reaction (emotional) is very different. The opposite may also occur; one person related to me that emotionally she is attracted to polyamory, but intellectually she is unsure.

Some people, when they have one loving partner, simply aren't interested in seeking others in addition, even after many years. Some people, when their partners gently and lovingly let it be known that they would like to explore possible emotional and sexual intimacy with someone else openly and honestly, experience fear, which can range anywhere from mild discomfort to major panic.

Whether you personally find polyamory to be the only way to live, or an impossible way to live, or something between, for yourself or your partner or both, depends largely on features of your personality. In short, polyamory is not for everyone.

No correlation with strength of bond. Whether polyamory will work well for you—whether you feel personally comfortable with a polyamorous lifestyle—is *not* a matter of how strongly you form loving bonds with someone else. It is unrelated to whether you are an extrovert or introvert. It is not a matter of whether you take the one you love into your deepest heart, or alternatively you take a cavalier attitude, saying to yourself, "Oh well, if I lose him/her, I'll just look for someone else, and meanwhile I'll get along living alone for a while." There is no apparent correlation between how strongly one forms loving bonds and whether that person identifies with polyamory or monamory.

No correlation with the homosexuality/heterosexuality spectrum. Gays and lesbians can be either polyamorous or monamorous, as can heterosexuals and bisexuals.

The concept of a monamorous bisexual may seem self-contradictory at first. Doesn't being bisexual mean being attracted to at least one person of each gender? No, some bisexuals find themselves attracted to *only one person at a time,* and that person may be of either gender. However, a great many bisexuals are also polyamorous.

At least in the polyamory community, bisexuality *appears* to be much more common among women than among men. That said, "appearances" in this case might hide another difference: Bi women appear to be typically more willing to be out about their bisexuality than are bi men, and this could inflate the apparent numbers of bi women compared to bi men. (Here is yet another unanswered sociological question.)

Orientation or choice? While there are many relationship practices and skills that are important for success in living polyamorously, following these practices will not guarantee you happiness living polyamorously.

1.04

We must also look at whether monamory or polyamory is an orientation or a choice for you.

The situation here is analogous to the question considered in earlier times as to how to "cure" homosexuality, when homosexuality was considered to be a psychological aberration. Psychotherapeutic attempts were made to "teach" lesbians and gays how to be happy loving someone of the other gender. No matter how much the homosexuals theoretically "learned" in the therapist's office, hetero bonding just was not in their nature.

Gays and lesbians in former times often actually married (someone of the other gender, that being the only option open), because it was socially expected of them or urged on them by their therapists, clergy, or family, but the results were usually disastrous. No doubt many still do.

Analogous to the spectrum of homosexuality to heterosexuality (sexual orientation), with degrees of bisexuality between, there *may* be a continuous spectrum of *orientation* towards either polyamory or monamory, with degrees between in which one can be happy with either kind of relationship ("biamorous"). Indications of an innate orientation are seen in the fact that some people (including this author) have identified with polyamorous attitudes since puberty, while others have always seemed just as strongly inclined to have only one mate at a time.

Whether the tendency toward polyamory or monamory is an innate orientation or is a deep-seated personality trait based on childhood experiences and other influences is by no means established at this writing, so to avoid misleading terminology, for now let's refer to this spectrum (whether innate or conditioned) as "number tendency" (a somewhat awkward term, yes, but it'll do for now). Just as a bisexual can enjoy a sexual relationship with someone of either gender, some people—

those who are biamorous—can be happy in either a monamorous or polyamorous loving relationship, while others simply *need* either pure monamory or pure polyamory in order to be happy in their love life. It may well be that number tendency is innate, or virtually so, in some people, and a matter of choice for others.

What feels right to you? Where are you on the spectrum of number tendency? Ask yourself: "When I have a strong loving relationship with someone, and it has gone beyond the phase of initial intense excitement ('new relationship energy'), do I lose interest in developing a romantic or sexual relationship with anyone else, or do I still sometimes find others attractive and sexy without losing any of the strength of my feelings for my existing partner?"

Can you change? If "number tendency" is innate, that would suggest that where you find yourself on that spectrum—how you answered that question above—is something fixed and unchangeable. In some cases this may be true, as also for sexual orientation, but the catch is that one may self-identify one way based on inadequate self-knowledge, without having experienced another way. So for example, a woman may have experienced sex only with other women and thus calls herself a lesbian; but, if she tries sex with a caring male friend, she may decide that she does also enjoy that, at least occasionally, and so she may change her sexual orientation category to "bisexual". A person may never have experienced polyamory, but, upon trying it, may find that they are comfortable with it, at least to some degree.

Think outside the box. Mainstream culture indoctrinates us into thinking that the only successful or "right" way to relate romantically and sexually is one at a time, "forsaking all others until death do you part"—just as it used to claim that the only "right" loving combination was one man and one woman (and some segments still do assert that).

Your choice. But it's your life—the most intimate aspect of your life—so the choice belongs to you and to no one else. If you think that polyamory is something that *might* be satisfying for you—if you're unattached, try it. If you're part of a couple, discuss it with your partner, and decide if the two of you want to try it together.

If after discussion you or your partner, but *not both* of you, are interested in trying the experiment, remember that there are many successful "poly/mono" couples, in which one partner is poly while the other prefers a monamorous life, but the mono partner accepts this difference between them, and the poly partner in turn works diligently to keep his/her mono partner assured that their own relationship remains primary. (See Section 2.08 about poly/mono relationships.)

1.05. *Finding suitable partners.*

The task of finding one or more others with whom to form a polyamorous relationship is in some ways no different from what any single person in mainstream society faces in finding a compatible mate; in other ways, there are differences.

If you are single and looking for one person with whom to form a primary polyamorous dyad, you naturally want to find someone compatible with you in the important ways—and, for you, of course one of those ways will be similar views about polyamory.

If you are single and hoping to connect with a couple or larger group, or if you are a couple or group seeking to add one or more other primary partners, the fundamental factors affecting compatibility remain unchanged, but in addition you will need to consider how *all* the people involved feel about the various factors of compatibility.

Because polyamory is a minority way of handling relationships, there is some temptation for poly people, even for those with some experience with relationships and their problems, when we find an available poly person, to leap for joy, throw caution to the wind, and rush ahead with grand ideas for forming a poly couple or triad or quad, etc., before we really know enough about potential bumps down that road if we do form a primary partnership with that person or those people. (I speak from experience!) One can have a wonderful, exciting secondary relationship while totally ignoring factors that would wreck an attempt to promote the relationship to primary status.

So the good news is that we can still really enjoy ourselves with a secondary-level dating relationship, while we let some time pass to get a better idea of how suitable the person(s) would or would not be as primary mates. In addition to time, we can do a "trial run" at living together—preferably for several months continuously, or at least for weekends or weeks, as the rest of life permits.

Let's say you've just met someone, and at first blush, as you and they have talked about things you have in common, they seem to show some promise as a new mate for you (or for both of you or all of you). Or you may have been dating this person for a while, but so far you haven't really gotten into discussing some of these factors that would become relevant only if you really lived together. How do you even know what to ask?

Appendix C, the "Quick Quirk Quotient Questionnaire", is designed to help in that regard, by suggesting a number of areas of life where each of us tends to have personal preferences one way or the other about how we live. It certainly is not exhaustive, but it should cover many or most of the significant questions that each of you really needs to think about if you're considering whether to move in together.

1.06. *Experimenting with polyamory as a couple.*

If you have no experience with open relationships. This section assumes that one or both of you have no prior experience with open relationships of any sort, including swinging. If you are experienced swingers, see section 1.07.

Set a time limit. In the stage of discussion and experimentation for a couple new to open relationships, a good tactic is to put a time limit on the experiment, say, two or three or six months, whatever feels comfortable for both of you. Agree that you will revisit the question after the trial period, or sooner if either of you wishes. Mark the date of expiration of this trial period on your appointment calendar so you don't forget.

The time limit is one way of assuring each other that your own relationship remains primary, foremost in your priorities; anything that gets in the way of that or threatens it must be put aside if a resolution or a way around the obstacle cannot be found.

If concerns or questions arise before the trial period expires, of course work through them, lovingly, candidly, thoroughly. (See Chapter 7 about resolving issues.)

Even if things seem to go well during the trial period, do go back when the time limit is reached and discuss again the fundamental question of whether to add polyamory to your relationship, based on your experience to date, and what variation of polyamory you will follow. Each of you needs to find out how the other feels—completely. Of course the two of you can set an additional trial period if you wish. If you decide to continue with polyamory, the two of you may decide at this point to fine-tune your agreement about how you will do it.

Unless both of you agree to continue after the time limit, then the experiment is ended; the two of you will continue your relationship as sexually exclusive (monamorous), according to your prior vow or agreement. This means that if you or your primary partner have "put your toes in the water" with a budding new secondary relationship, and then you and your primary partner decide that the existence of that secondary relationship is just too threatening to your primary relationship, and the two of you cannot resolve those issues, then it is important to the health of the primary relationship to break off the secondary relationship, at least in its sexual aspect.

Of course breaking off with a secondary in that situation should be done lovingly, with consideration and empathy. If you enter into a secondary relationship during this sort of trial period, honesty and integrity says that the secondary partner should know about the trial period from the start, knowing that the outcome of the experiment might require breaking off the secondary relationship.

Moratoriums. Even if you and your primary partner decide that the experiment has worked well and you're both content to embark on polyamory as your ongoing lifestyle, problems may arise later, either regarding a particular secondary or in some aspect of your primary relationship having nothing to do with polyamory or that particular secondary partner. If such problems do arise, you and your primary partner may wish to consider placing a "moratorium" on secondary relationships so you can focus all your energies and attention on resolving the issue that has arisen. Like the initial trial period, I suggest that the two of you agree on a set period of time, after which you decide together whether to lift the moratorium or extend it.

Moratoriums early in a primary relationship (for building that relationship) are discussed in more detail in section 6.04; moratoriums when issues arise later in a relationship are discussed in section 7.13.

1.07. Moving from swinging to polyamory.

Is swinging the only game in town? Many couples and individuals have become involved in swinging as the only known alternative to mainstream sexual exclusivity (monamory). They feel hemmed in by the mainstream default prohibition against multiple sexual partners, and they figure that as long as they are open and honest with the ones closest to them, and if they proceed responsibly, then adding new sex partners can only add variety and fun to their life. They know that many couples have been active swingers for many years, evidently quite happy in their own relationship as well as with their swinging friends.

After a while, as with any interest group, many swingers will form friendships, some of them perhaps quite close, strong, and loving. When they go to one of their swing club's sex parties, they keep seeking out their friends, fending off other invitations to the back rooms as best they can. Whether or not they form close friendships, they may come to feel that they would like to see more attention to emotional connectedness to go with the sex.

Overlap. As we noted in section 1.02, swinging and polyamory shade into each other with no clear boundary, the differences being mostly a matter of emphasis—recreational sex that may include warm, caring feelings, or multiple loving relationships that can include sex—and sometimes the sex in polyamory can come rather quickly. So, you may think of yourself as a swinger who likes personal connections more than do most other swingers. The reverse is certainly also possible: Someone may come to open relationships via polyamory, but then feel that most polyamorists are just too slow to get it on!

If you are in the latter group, you may identify better with swinging than with polyamory. We wish you success in finding what you're looking for, and you'll still be welcome to visit with us in the polyamory community whenever you would like. There is no reason you cannot be active in both communities.

If you think of yourself as a swinger but you find that you are often not much interested in sharing sex with someone new until you've gotten to know and care for them to some degree—if you would rather have one or a few good, warm relationships rather than constant new faces in bed with you—then you may find that you identify more with polyamory.

There are also people who like to stay in the cross-over area, comfortable both with multiple emotional relationships in the style of polyamory and with recreational sex in the swinging style.

Making the transition. Shifting from swinging to the polyamory community (or vice versa) should be relatively easy compared to the transition from monamory to any sexually open lifestyle. Because of the differences noted in section 1.02, however, if you are an experienced swinger now exploring the polyamory community, you should be alert to differences in expected conduct—especially with regard to sex. At a swingers' sex party, it is normal and accepted for one person to invite another to share sex after an introduction and only a few minutes of light chatting. Among polyamorists, an approach this fast would often be seen as quite boorish. In polyamory, both parties may indeed feel a fast mutual sexual attraction—and there's nothing wrong with letting someone know that you find yourself quite attracted to them—but polyamorists usually develop their acquaintance with someone more before one suggests sex to the other.

Similarly, if you as an experienced swinger join a local poly group and introduce yourself to the group in person at an event or via the group's email discussion list, or if you place a personal ad on a poly-focused ad site, it is gauche to emphasize things like your penis or breast size, sexual endurance, and the like. Polyamorists as a rule would rather hear first about what you're like in your mind, heart, and spirit, and what hobbies and recreations you enjoy. This does not mean that polyamorists do not have preferences about body dimensions, height, weight, and other physical characteristics. But we want to come to like you as a person first; otherwise your physical characteristics and your prowess in bed are not likely to matter much to us.

So introduce yourself and let us get to know you!

1.08. Expressing your initial interest to someone.

How do I let a polyamorous person know that I'm interested? In the single world, most of us learn fairly early on, usually in adolescence, how to let someone know that we find them attractive and we'd like to have a date so we can start to get to know them better. Based largely on gender role stereotypes, or just on what feels comfortable for us personally, either we learn to ask another single person for a date, or by hints and body language we let the other person know that we'd like them to ask for a date.

But no matter how comfortable and adept you become at directly or indirectly initiating single-to-single dating relationships, that all gets turned upside-down in the world of polyamory, where the object of your interest, as likely as not, is already married or has a committed or serious partner. As likely as not, you have someone in your life as well.

Whether you are single or in a couple relationship yourself, let's suppose you find another polyamorous person who is interesting, but they are in a committed relationship. Do you approach this person in the same way as if you both were single? Is this person's primary partner going to fly into an uproar at you for daring to try to get something going, as is normal and expected in mainstream society?

Polyamorists have their own individual preferences about how to receive this sort of expression of interest, for themselves or for their primary partners. It's a fairly safe assumption, though, that if you know that a couple is polyamorous, then it's okay to express your interest in exploring the possibilities with one of them, or both of them, as long as you do so in a respectful manner, not crudely or brutishly, in the same way as if both of you were single. The person you are interested in may decline you equally politely, with something like, "Sorry, I like you as a friend, but I'm not interested in developing anything more intimate with you"—again, in a way similar to the dynamics between two single people. Or, they may let you know that they are also interested, and then you can take it from there.

Poly couples (or larger primary groups, such as triads or quads) also have varying preferences or agreements about how they may individually form new secondary relationships. See section 2.03 for details about that. Here, we are looking at the other side of that coin, as you let someone in a couple (or larger group) know that you are interested in exploring the possibilities with them.

Because of those variations in how couples handle that situation, you may be told, "Okay, but my spouse/partner would like to meet you first, and then he/she and I will have to decide between us whether it's okay for me to date you." Or, "Okay, and I will let my spouse/partner know that you and I are planning a date, or that we've had a date." Or simply, "Okay."

If the other person responds with something like, "Okay, but I'll have to call you; don't call me because my partner might answer," this is a red flag! See section 3.02.

If the object of your interest is in a couple relationship, even if the other person does not tell you that they must get agreement first from their primary partner, it is a good idea for you to *offer* to meet the other person's primary (if you don't already know them), since this will demonstrate your intention to be open and honest about your secondary involvement. Meeting your interest's primary also assures you, of course, that your interest is not trying to do something behind their primary's back.

What if you don't know whether someone in a couple is polyamorous? If you become interested in someone, and you know that they are part of a couple, but you do not know if they have a polyamorous agreement between them, you can still show your interest respectfully, although of

1.08

course there will be the additional step of finding out if their relationship is open to dating others.

Even if you learn that their couple relationship is on the traditional, monamorous model, you could still express your interest and raise the possibility of a closer involvement, though you will need to tread very carefully in this situation. In this case, in letting the other person know that you are attracted and you would like to get to know them better, it is important to stress that you do not want to do anything contrary to their own agreement or vows with their spouse or partner; you do not want to do anything in secret. If the other person is also interested in you, but says that they and their partner have not considered allowing outside relationships, then you could suggest that they talk about it between themselves and decide whether to allow it, then get back to you. It would be good for you to offer to meet your interest's primary (if you do not already know each other).

If your interest says that they will bring the question up with their primary, then there is nothing further you can do until they make their decision one way or the other, except to jog the other person's memory occasionally to let them know that you are still interested, and perhaps to ask now and then about the status of discussions. When a couple is first considering whether to open their relationship to polyamory-style outside relationships, they may feel the need to move slowly and carefully, and of course you will not want to make them feel that you are rushing them. (See section 1.09 if you are in that couple yourself and someone expresses interest in you.)

Communicating with your interest's primary partner. This area, too, goes contrary to all the conditioning that we receive in mainstream culture, and so it may take a while to become comfortable communicating frankly with the spouse or primary partner of the person that you're interested in. Here, too, preferences vary among individual polyamorists, so it is best to ask the person you are interested in, first, whether or how much their primary partner would want to talk with you about these things.

Let's suppose you have expressed your interest to someone in a committed polyamorous couple, and the other person has returned your interest, and you then ask about speaking directly with their primary partner. If the answer is, "Sure, we welcome complete communication," it is still a good idea to ask your interest's primary about their comfort level before launching into questions or commentary about very intimate topics. Here is an example from personal experience to illustrate my point.

My primary partner, Deborah, and I together met a man at a restaurant gathering of our local polyamory group. He let us both know, hesitantly, that he was attracted to Deborah, and that his girlfriend (who was not present that evening) might also be interested in getting to know both of us. Both of them, he said, were totally comfortable with the idea of polyamory, but both had little experience so far, and he was not sure how to approach us. Deborah let him know that she also found him interesting, and so, yes, she would also like to get better acquainted with him. We both told him that we would be glad to meet his girlfriend as well, if she chose to meet us.

The next day, he phoned our home, and it happened that Deborah was away, so he and I chatted. He again hesitantly asked if I was willing to talk with him some about what the possibilities might be. As I replied to him, it happens that Deborah and I are both completely comfortable (unlike some polyamorists) in talking with secondaries or potential new secondaries for the other of us, and so I answered his questions about how and when we might all arrange to meet in a restaurant to get better acquainted, and also (if we decide to go further) the sorts of things that Deborah and I both enjoy sexually. I feel that this sort of conversation,

1.08

while not necessary, can sometimes smooth the way for all concerned and avoid exploring dead-end paths. For example, our new friend and I might have discovered that his interests for sexual activities did not overlap at all with Deborah's, in which case we would have known right there that there would be no point trying to develop a sexual component to the relationship, although of course we could all remain nonsexual friends in that case.

Of course, when you ask your new interest about speaking with their primary, you may be told something like, "Well, we have agreed to be open to secondary relationships, but we don't want to share any specific information with each other about any outside relationships." In other words, they have a "don't ask, don't tell" relationship. This precludes your being able to talk with your interest's primary—or, if you do, it precludes your mentioning anything that would reveal your interest in developing a secondary relationship with their primary. (See section 6.07 for more about "don't ask, don't tell" relationships.)

Polyamorous couples have a whole spectrum of degrees of sharing and communication between them, between "don't ask, don't tell" and "anything goes, and we tell each other everything."

Although "don't ask, don't tell" relationships are considered to fit within the parameters of "openness and honesty" (because no one is being deceived), proceed with caution if someone that you are interested in tells you that they have such an arrangement with their partner. Since you cannot directly verify the truth of what you are told (because you cannot talk to the other partner), about your only recourse is to satisfy yourself that the person you are interested in is truthful by nature, so that they are deceiving neither you nor their partner. In some cases, if you know the other partner anyway, you might be able to engage in a *general* conversation about their poly lifestyle (without revealing your personal interest in their partner), finding out how the two of them handle poly arrangements in general, while sharing your own preferences and practices.

If you start such a general conversation about polyamory with your interest's primary, and you ask in general how that person and their partner manage their poly life, and if that person then responds with surprise that they are not polyamorous—well, there you have your answer. The person you are interested in has lied to you. Also see section 3.07.

1.09. *If a committed person receives an expression of interest.*

Let's say you are married, or in a comparable committed relationship, and someone lets you know that they are interested in getting to know you better, explicitly or implicitly suggesting that they might want to develop a secondary-level sexual relationship with you. (If this person is bisexual or gay/lesbian, and you or your primary are also, the expression of interest might be for both of you.)

If you and your primary are already polyamorous, or have agreed to try it. As section 2.03 indicates, it is up to the individual preferences of you and your primary partner how you arrange secondary relationships. You and your primary may prefer for both of you to get to know a potential new secondary before anything intimate develops, or you may prefer for each of you not to involve yourselves as much or at all in the other's secondary relationships.

Let's say that you are in a committed relationship, your primary and you already practice polyamory (or you're open to try it), and someone expresses an interest in you and/or your partner, or another couple expresses interest. How do you handle this? In this situation, you are on the receiving end of what I described in section 1.08, where you want to express your interest in a person who is in a committed relationship.

The first time that someone expresses interest in one of you, the situation may feel awkward both to you and your partner. This awkwardness is normal, since this kind of inquiry goes against traditional social conditioning that, once a committed couple relationship is formed, there should be no further intimacy with anyone else.

Don't rush. If this would be your first venture into polyamorous intimacy, whether only one of you in the primary couple or both of you might develop this potential secondary relationship, it would be a good idea to go slowly and cautiously, rather than yielding quickly to the call of your hormones. There are at least two reasons for this.

For one, you may be glad later if you develop a nonsexual friendship with this other person or couple for a while, to get to know them better, and see if the mutual interest in something more continues, or was a flash in the pan. This will let the two of you, as primary partners, check in with each other frequently about your feelings about the situation as it develops. If either of you is having misgivings, maybe some feelings of jealousy, now is the time to bring those feelings out! It is far better not to venture into multiple relationships, if that is not what really suits the temperaments of both of you, than to plunge ahead and then have to try to repair damage to your relationship.

If either of you does discover feelings of jealousy when you contemplate a possible outside involvement, the good news is that jealousy is learned, and so it can be unlearned. Jealousy is not a fundamental emotion, but results from deeper feelings, generally involving fear and personal insecurities. If the jealousy is fairly substantial, you may find it helpful to seek professional psychotherapy to get to the bottom of it and grow beyond it. If you do overcome your jealousy, you will benefit as a person, and as a couple, in ways far broader than just the issue of jealousy itself. Jealousy is discussed in more detail in section 7.05.

The other reason for going slow at first is that judging other people's characters is a learned skill; we get better at it with practice and with personal emotional and spiritual development. Earlier in adult life, we often find that our initial assessments of someone else turn out to be not very accurate after we get to know them better. With greater experience, we more often find that our initial impressions were correct. So, especially if you are now in your earlier adult years, you may want to give yourself more time to become more sure that this other person is someone that you want to share a bed with, and other parts of your life.

When you were single and unattached, perhaps you were less concerned about the character of someone you might share sex with. If you enjoyed the person's company momentarily, that was good enough. But now that you are part of a committed couple, negative repercussions from a hasty sexual liaison could rock the boat in your primary relationship.

So take it in steps, and talk it over with your partner at each step of the way.

~ 2 ~

Varieties of Polyamory

Contents:
2.01. Many varieties.
2.02. Polyamory for the single person.
2.03. Polyamory for couples.
2.04. Polyamory for triads and larger groups.
2.05. Clans, tribes, and communities.
2.06. Line marriages.
2.07. Intentional communities.
2.08. The poly/mono mixed relationship.
2.09. The poly/swinger mixed relationship.
2.10. Relevance of the term "secondary".
2.11. From the perspective of the secondary.
2.12. Sexual alphabet soup.

♥ ♥ ♥

2.01. Many varieties.

Some in the polyamory community say that there are as many different varieties of polyamory as there are polyamorists. It is certainly true that the basic notion of polyamory can be expressed in many different ways in real life, but at least we can identify some categories and common variations.

As section 1.01 points out, there are also limits to the concept of polyamory. See that section for a discussion of what polyamory is not, as well as what it is.

The sections of this chapter will look at polyamory for the single person, the couple, the triad, etc., to larger groups.

2.02. Polyamory for the single person.

By "single person" here I mean someone who is emotionally unattached—who not only is not married but is not living with nor dating anyone in an emotionally involved relationship, and not in a committed relationship.

The term could also include someone who is legally married but separated; that is, the marital relationship is no longer functional and has no emotional content. It could also include a married or committed person still living together with their spouse or partner in a lifeless relationship; this would be up to the individual to assess, and perhaps discuss with the partner. The key factor in the latter situation would be whether one partner would have any feelings about or reaction to the other partner pursuing a social life with one or more other people. That is, do you *both feel unattached* even though you're still under the same roof?

Just dating? It might seem that polyamory for the single person is really no different from ordinary dating. It's commonplace for a single person to have multiple dating partners. But if you are single and dating more than one, do you inform each dating partner that you date others?

Informing them all and giving each of them details of your other dating relationships may not be necessary, appropriate, or consistent with polyamory. It depends on the intensity of a given dating relationship—and of course there's no visible boundary between a more casual and a more involved dating relationship, so it's a judgment call.

As you become more involved with a given dating partner, it becomes steadily more important for you to let that person know about the existence of other dating partners. Some people, as they become more deeply involved in a dating relationship, will tacitly assume that the relationship is exclusive, unless they are informed otherwise. (It would be a *mistake* to make that kind of assumption, but people sometimes do, and that leads to hurt feelings and arguments.)

You may say to yourself, "Well, I never claimed to A that I'm *not* also dating B and C, so if A makes an assumption without actually asking, that's A's problem!" True enough, strictly speaking, but, again, you are cruising for stormy waters with A if by silence you allow A to make an unwarranted assumption and then A learns that they are not alone in your heart after all. As your relationship with A deepens, the situation becomes gradually more similar to that of someone who learns that their spouse has been having a secret "affair" (see section 1.01). These storms can be avoided, or at least greatly lessened, by keeping all of your dating partners informed, starting fairly early on, not only about the existence of other dating partners but about the general depth or seriousness of the other relationships. Talk to them, sooner rather than later, about your polyamorous relationship philosophy or orientation.

How to communicate with new acquaintances about your polyamorous nature or lifestyle is discussed in more detail in section 6.03.

Another way in which polyamory may be relevant to you as a single person is that you may come to consider one or more dating relationships to be "primary", that is, more important or central in your life, while other dating relationships are "secondary", less important.

Relationships with married or committed people. One sharp difference between nonpoly and poly dating for the single person is that polyamory allows you to pursue relationships with people who are married or similarly committed, as long as you do so with honesty and ethical concern for all. This means that you need to take into account your potential new lover's primary relationship and what expectations or agreements there are between those two primary partners.

See section 3.02 about the ethics of becoming sexually involved with someone who is married or committed. See section 2.11 about your own attitudes toward being in the role of secondary, whether you are unattached or are yourself in a committed relationship.

2.03. *Polyamory for couples.*

Emotionally dead couple relationships. See the first two paragraphs of section 2.02 if you are married or living with someone in a committed relationship, but you *both* consider that the relationship is no longer functional; that is, neither of you has feelings one way or the other about whether the other of you pursues a social life with other people.

Varieties of secondary relationship. If you are in a couple (marriage or other committed relationship), you and your partner may develop a secondary relationship together with an individual, or with another dyad, etc.; or either of you may want to form relationships as an individual with a single, a couple, etc., without involving the other primary partner. The two of you should discuss together in advance of any outside involvement whether you will be comfortable with one of you dating without the other, and, if so, how much information you want to share with each other and other details.

See Chapter 5 about the relationship agreement and Chapter 6 about communication techniques. See section 2.11 about the secondary relationship from the perspective of the secondary partner.

Both primaries dating together. This variation has the advantage that the two primary partners are doing something together, so neither will feel left out, and it adds to the shared couple experience. Threesome and foursome sex can be very exciting, if all parties are comfortable. (It may take a little getting used to, since we have to unlearn societal conditioning that sex "should" involve only two people and be done in privacy from others.)

A disadvantage of dating together as a couple could be the need to find a third person or another couple whom *both* primaries would enjoy dating together, and who would enjoy dating a couple.

Dating together as a couple could be a compromise position if either of the primaries is uncomfortable, potentially jealous, at the thought of the other primary dating someone else without them.

Dating separately. This variation gives greater flexibility in that one person finds another person to date, similar to dating among singles. There are new complexities, however, not present among singles.

How much of a say does one primary partner have in the other primary's outside dating companions or activities? This can vary from zero ("go out with whoever you want and have fun—just don't bring any diseases home") to veto power ("I want to meet the person first and agree with you in advance that you may spend time alone with them or share sex with them"). The primary couple should discuss this question and reach agreement before any potential new secondary relationships arise, and include that in their relationship agreement (see Chapter 5).

There are intermediate positions on the question between giving your partner *carte blanche* and holding veto power. You can agree to require meeting a potential new secondary for the other of you in advance, but then leave it to your partner's personal choice to continue, without veto power. You can agree to be informed in advance by telephone, email, online chat, etc., if physical separation makes advance meeting in person impractical. You can agree to inform each other as soon as practical *following* a first sexual involvement with a new secondary—say, the next day if practical. The latter two options are especially useful when one of the primaries is away, at a conference for example, and "clicks" with someone there.

2.03

Keeping each other informed. When one primary partner is carrying on a secondary relationship or is starting a new one, normally it is important to keep the other primary(-ies) well informed not just of the existence of the secondary relationship but of the intensity of feelings, any changes in its nature, and other details. However, some primary couples prefer (and agree) that they *do not want* detailed information about secondary relationships. The understanding could be along the lines that "we agree that either of us may have outside (secondary) sexual relationships, but we do not wish to know of actual relationships that may exist" (a "don't ask, don't tell" policy); or, "we agree to inform each other of the existence of any secondary relationship, but we do not wish to meet the person, know what is done, or know any other details."

This sort of arrangement may be workable, but should be pursued very carefully and attentively, because an unwillingness to know details may mask a conscious or subconscious discomfort by one of the primaries with allowing their partner to have any sort of secondary relationship. One primary partner may agree to allow secondary relationships with the private motive of "not rocking the boat" in the primary relationship. Not expressing such dissatisfactions can cause more damage than "rocking the boat" and talking them out, because the dissatisfactions accumulate and balloon over time, eventually exploding into the open, often in a very unpleasant way. If such discomfort is openly acknowledged early on, however, then this sort of restricted disclosure can be healthy and positive—but be careful, nonetheless; you should both look carefully into all those cobwebby recesses of your own mind and your partner's mind with a good flashlight.

Communications (and consequences for not communicating) are treated more fully in Chapter 6. Chapter 4 includes a discussion of safe sex considerations with secondaries—condom use; when fluid-bondedness with a secondary can be considered; what to do if a condom breaks or slips off with a secondary, or if a secondary is diagnosed with an STD.

2.04. *Polyamory for triads and larger groups.*

Also see Chapter 9 for a more detailed discussion of the dynamics of triads and larger committed groups. See section 2.06 about line marriages and section 2.07 about intentional communities.

The discussion in this section is equally valid for triads and for primary groups larger than three. In this section I will use the term "multiple family" to refer to triads, quads, pentads, etc.

Polyamorous dynamics within the multiple family. All of the dynamics, principles, relationship skills, etc., that are important for keeping a couple together and happy apply also (even more so, usually) in a multiple family. In addition, however, there are a number of sexual and nonsexual dynamics that arise in a multiple family but that are absent in couples.

Sexual dynamics. The sexual dynamics within a multiple family will obviously depend on the sexual orientations of the individual members. In the most common triad configuration, with two partners of one gender and the third partner of the other gender, sex in all three twosome combinations will occur only if both partners who share gender are bisexual. Otherwise, the multiple family will be a sexual "V", with the partner whose gender is not shared at the angle of the "V".

Other combinations of orientations can also result in a "V". One triad known to the author involves a hetero man, a lesbian woman, and a bisexual woman. Clearly the man and the lesbian are each sexual only with the bi woman, who is at the angle of the "V".

However, a "V" does not mean that the triad cannot enjoy threesome sex. As one example, let's assume two hetero men and a woman. The two men can enjoy giving pleasure simultaneously to the woman, who can give plenty of attention to both of her male partners simultaneously. Many women greatly enjoy receiving the attention of two men at the same time.

A sexual "V" also does not prevent a full, three-sided *emotional* relationship among all partners of the triad.

Similar dynamics apply in multiple families larger than a triad.

Nonsexual dynamics. Interactions between members of a multiple family can occur that are impossible in a couple. In a couple, if a difference of views arises, and if the partners fail to reach agreement after some discussion, they may simply decide to "agree to disagree"; "you have your opinion and I have mine." However, in a triad or larger, the possibility of *majority and minority* arises. The consequences of this are discussed in Chapter 7.

Secondary relationships for members of multiple families. In addition to the polyamorous aspects *within* a multiple family, the family needs to consider the additional question of whether the primary partners may engage in secondary relationships *outside* the family. The practice by a multiple family of restricting sex to those within the group is called *polyfidelity;* the adjective form is *polyfidelitous.*

When a multiple family makes the decision either to adopt polyfidelity or not, that decision should become part of their group relationship agreement (see Chapter 5). All the partners in a newly formed multiple family may feel no interest in pursuing secondary relationships, but it is still a good idea to discuss this question and place the decision in the relationship agreement, in order to avoid surprises and strife caused by assumptions and misunderstandings if one or more of the partners later wants to develop a secondary relationship, or (even worse) gets involved first and runs it by their partners later.

Reasons for polyfidelity. A multiple family might choose polyfidelity for reasons similar to why a couple chooses monamory (twosome sexual exclusivity). That is, given the complexity of the relationship dynamics within the primary group, the group may decide to avoid the still more complex dynamics that arise when secondary relationships are added to the mix. A polyfidelitous group may also prefer the increased confidence of being free of STDs, once they have all tested disease-free themselves. Or, it may simply be that none in the group are interested in developing relationships outside the primary group.

Allowing secondary relationships. The dynamics and questions surrounding secondary relationships that arise for a multiple family are similar to those for a couple (see section 2.02), although (not surprisingly) there can be more complexity and variations in a group of three or more. One member of a multiple family, or two of them, or all of them, might develop a secondary relationship with one other person, or another couple, or triad, etc. In a multiple family, more different opinions are possible about all the questions that arise in polyamorous couples, such as *carte blanche* vs. veto power or something between, how to keep each other informed, whether a given outside person would make a good secondary partner for one of them, and all the rest.

2.05. *Clans, tribes, and communities.*

When a primary polyamorous family grows to more than about four or five adult members, things tend to blur. Especially with larger groups, members may not all live under the same roof or on the same land (as an "intentional community"—see section 2.06). Some emotional relationships between pairs of members may be felt to be "more primary" than others, or less so. Some nominally "secondary" partners of some members may develop closer ties with one or more members of the group than with other members, frequently sharing meals and activities, sleeping over, etc. Some members may be polyamorously linked with other members, some not.

In short, as an intimate group grows, its dynamics gradually come to resemble that of organizations or communities in general, acquiring new members and losing others, having varying roles and degrees of personal involvement and leadership in the group, etc.

A primary family of this size is one way to resolve possible imbalances felt when there is a large age difference between primary partners. These imbalances are felt most acutely when there are only two or three primary partners; as the size of the primary family increases, the more likely it is that there will be one or more other partners fairly close in age to any other.

Nomenclature reflects the blurring of distinction between family and organization. Members may feel that the terms "primary" and "secondary" are not very meaningful for their group. The group itself will probably not call itself by a term reflecting their exact number, such as "pentad", "hexad", or "heptad", but will use a looser term, such as "intimate network", "clan", "tribe", "family", or "community".

Also see section 2.06 about line marriages.

2.06. *Line marriages.*

In the mid 1960s and 1970s the science fiction author Robert H. Heinlein had some of the characters in his literary works living a variety of innovative lifestyles, including polyamory (though of course he didn't call it that, since that word would not be coined for another two decades). One variation of polyamory envisioned by Heinlein was the "line marriage"—and he did coin that term.

Some in the modern polyamory community have put that fictional line marriage concept into real-life practice, including the term.

A line marriage starts with a couple, triad, quad, etc.—a dyad or a multi-adult primary-level committed group of a sort familiar to us in the 21st century. Over a span of years, as older group members eventually die off, new, younger adults join the group, maintaining an approximately stable size and allowing the group to continue its existence indefinitely, potentially for centuries.

A line marriage could be thought of as a type of "clan" or "tribe" (see section 2.05). There is no typical size to line marriages, but, as you can imagine, a mature line marriage could typically entail half a dozen to a dozen or more partners, spanning the entire adult age range. As mentioned in section 2.05, a group of this size could include some twosome partnerships that are emotionally closer or deeper than others; some pairs may share sex and some not.

2.07. Intentional communities.

See the Glossary entry (Appendix B) for "community" for a definition of "intentional community".

Intentional communities (ICs) are not necessarily polyamorous in their internal relationship structure. Some are 100% polyamorous (by design or happenstance), some partially so, some not at all. Most, though not all, are at least accepting of open polyamory among their members.

Regardless of the extent to which a specific IC accepts polyamory, the interpersonal dynamics of any IC resemble those of a polyamorous family in many ways, including mutual respect and trust, honesty, integrity, common purposes and goals, open and thorough communication, working together on tasks, decision-making and conflict resolution, etc. For this reason, many polyamorous people are drawn to join or form ICs, and many IC members are drawn to polyamory.

For couples in which one or both partners are unwilling to consider living polyamorously, life in an IC can offer many of the same benefits (and challenges) as polyamory, minus the sexual diversity. Benefits include greater social interaction with people who may share one's specific interests, recreations, etc., more than one's partner; help with daily life maintenance like childcare, shopping, cooking, home maintenance, and the like. Challenges (which could also be benefits!) include the necessity to confront one's personal "growing edges" and heal and grow in those areas, in order to function smoothly in close association with a number of other people; time demands for meetings; some loss of personal privacy unless steps are taken to protect that.

Like polyamory, one could say that there about as many different ways of living in an IC as there are ICs. Many are in a rural setting with enough land area to grow part or all of their own food. Many (commonly calling themselves "co-housing communities") are in urban or suburban areas, and consist of a large house or several adjacent houses in which the members live. Many (often calling themselves "ecovillages") are especially concerned to live in an ecologically (environmentally) responsible way, minimizing use of nonrenewable resources and using renewable resources sustainably.

Both urban and rural communities (more commonly with the rural ones) are often partially or entirely "off the grid" electrically; i.e., they do not buy electrical power, or not all of it, from the public electric power network, or grid, but generate their own using photovoltaic panels, wind turbines, mini-hydroelectric plants, or other technology.

See section A.03 in Appendix A for contact information about the IC umbrella organization, Fellowship for Intentional Community. Also see section 9.05 about the overlap area between a large polyamorous family and an IC.

2.08. *The poly/mono mixed relationship.*

Sometimes one member of an established, committed dyad decides they strongly wish to live polyamorously (they are reluctant to "compromise away" their poly orientation), while their partner simply has no interest in maintaining multiple loving relationships. Is this relationship doomed? Must they struggle to find agreement on a common lifestyle, or else sadly give up and go their separate ways?

The news here is good. Mixed "poly/mono relationships", as they are called, do exist and do work. (And no, it isn't always the guy who wants to branch out while his female partner wants to stay home.)

How to make a poly/mono relationship work. The first necessary ingredient, not surprisingly, is plenty of love, trust, and good will on both sides, generating the desire to find a way of life for themselves that satisfies each of them individually as well as nurturing their couple relationship.

If there are other issues. If the couple has other issues pending between them, they need to work to find resolution to these if at all possible, before attempting to establish themselves as a poly/mono couple. Attempting to add yet another difference or complication between them (one of them pursuing secondary relationships, the other not, even if by mutual agreement) could create stresses and instability in their relationship.

If the relationship is solid. If love and trust are well grounded between the two partners, then the mechanics of making a poly/mono relationship work are really not so difficult. The partners agree that the poly-oriented partner will keep the monamorous partner informed (to the extent that the latter desires) of the existence and conduct of any secondary relationships, similar to how it is done when both partners of a dyad are polyamorous. It would be good to place the details of this understanding into a relationship agreement (see Chapter 5). Of course the relationship agreement will also contain specific provisions, same as for a poly-poly couple, about the safe sex standards that the poly/mono couple have agreed on together.

It is also *very* important for the poly partner (P) to give *continual and strong* reinforcement, in word and deed, to their mono partner (M) that P keeps M first and foremost in P's heart, and that everything else must yield to the preeminent importance of keeping their own relationship sound, loving, and mutually enriching. This reassurance is essential for enabling M to continue feeling satisfied and confident that P's secondary relationships will not pose a threat to their own primary relationship.

M, for their part, being thus reassured by P, agrees to support P lovingly, while of course being careful always to express their own feelings and desires in the relationship.

One word of caution is in order here. Once or twice I've heard of couples in which one partner wants the privilege of poly-style secondary relationships for himself or herself but is unwilling to allow the same privilege for their partner. This *should* be too obvious to need mentioning, but this would *not* be a legitimate variation of "poly/mono", because of the blatant sexism, possessiveness, control, or whatever is working here. What's good for the goose is good for the gander (or vice versa). A genuine poly/mono relationship is one in which the mono partner *chooses* not to pursue poly-style secondary relationships; the exclusiveness is not thrust upon them unwillingly by their primary partner who wants the privilege of multiple relationships to be one-sided.

2.09. *The poly/swinger mixed relationship.*

It can also happen, of course, that both members of a couple would like the freedom to pursue other sexual involvements, but one likes looser, less emotionally involved sex with many partners, along the swinging model (see section 1.02), while the other prefers to limit their outside sex to one or a few secondary partners with whom there is substantial emotional connection and mutual caring, polyamory-style.

Whether this is a problem for such a couple, if they are male/female, might depend on which partner is swinging-oriented and which is more polyamorous. Men and women are usually treated differently regarding solo participation in swinging organizations and activities. If a married man shows interest in joining such a group alone, he will be politely asked to bring his wife to the orientation session; otherwise he will not be welcome. If a married woman inquires alone, she probably will also be asked at least to get something signed by her husband showing that he's aware and consents to her participation, and maybe he'll be asked to show up at an orientation meeting with his wife, but then she will probably be welcomed into the group alone, as will an unmarried woman. (A swinging group may or may not try to concern itself with the gray area of unmarried cohabiting relationships, with their wide range of emotional commitment.)

Between the two partners themselves, the mutual understanding that they need to reach would resemble that in the poly/mono relationship, described in section 2.08. Each would need to recognize the legitimacy of their partner's preferences regarding outside relationships. They should prepare a relationship agreement (Chapter 5) setting out what they have agreed, and giving special attention to the safe sex provisions, since the swinging partner will inevitably be exposing them both to additional health risk.

If it is the male partner who is swinging-oriented, he will probably not be welcome to join or attend group swinging activities alone (even if they have joined the group as a couple), as mentioned above. One option for him, with his primary's consent and if the group allows it, would be to join the swinging group with a different woman, one who is herself swinging-oriented. Another option is for his female primary to join and attend events (including sexual parties) with him; and, for the openly sexual events, she could try to cultivate especially warm relationships with one or a few others who regularly attend, so that she could limit her sexual attentions at the parties just to those few others, who would then approximate the poly concept of "secondary partners". Perhaps she would then be more comfortable with the knowledge that her partner has someone different in a back room at each party, if that is his preference.

If it is the female member of the poly-swinger couple who is swinging-oriented, the practicalities are simpler, since swinging groups tend to welcome women without a male companion, as noted. She can attend a swingers' party alone while her primary goes to his poker club or does his bagpipe practice when she doesn't have to listen, and both will be happy. Or he may decide to attend the parties with his partner to see if he can meet one or a few regular back-room partners, as when the genders are reversed.

Who knows, it could well happen that, after some experience in this manner, the swinging-oriented partner may also develop one or a few especially warm relationships within the group, so that he or she shifts their attitude more toward the polyamorous model; or maybe the polyamorist of the two will decide they enjoy more sex partners with less connectedness.

If one shifts one way while the other shifts the other way, I hope they both have a sense of humor!

2.10. Relevance of the term "secondary".

Some poly people, especially singles, feel that the terms "primary" and "secondary" don't fit well with their style of relating; they say, "But I care for all my partners; I don't want to rank them." It's fine if you simply prefer to keep any or all of your emotional and sexual partners on the same level; that's just a matter of preference.

Some people feel that the *term* "secondary" is demeaning or pejorative. This is not the case at all. It is simply a factual description for a partner or relationship that does take a lesser priority than another partner or relationship that is treated as "primary". If you are married or in a comparable committed relationship, then any other dating relationships that you or your primary partner may have will normally have to yield if there is any conflict in scheduling or in any other way that cannot be resolved.

You could choose to use some term other than "secondary" if you wish, but the fact remains that if you are in a committed relationship, you give precedence or priority to that relationship, so that other relationships must be held in a lesser position, by whatever term you choose to call it.

I use the terms "primary" and "secondary" freely, in this book and elsewhere, because I feel that they are the terms that best describe the concept, and I do not consider that the term "secondary" is at all demeaning or pejorative.

2.11. *From the perspective of the secondary.*

There are two ways that you can be in a secondary relationship. One is if you already have one or more primary partners, and a new relationship for you would be on a lesser level of involvement and commitment. (Your secondary partner in this case might or might not have their own primary partner(s).) The other way is if the other person has one or more primary partners, but you have none. Your own partnerless status here cannot change the fact that you will be a secondary with this other person—unless all agree to bring you into

2.11

your lover's primary group, forming a triad or larger multi-primary family.

Of course you may have a dating relationship that has these "secondary" characteristics even if you and the other person are both single (emotionally unattached). However, if neither you nor the other person is in a primary relationship, then this dating relationship is not *called* "secondary", since there is nothing for it to be secondary to. (See section 2.02.)

Some emotionally unattached people lead busy lives involving their career, children, hobbies, recreations, dates, etc.; they like it that way; and they just aren't interested in giving some of that up in order to invest the considerable time and effort required to build and maintain a *primary* relationship. If you are one such person, you might well prefer to keep all your relationships on the secondary level or dating level even if one dating relationship of yours might have the *potential* of being "promoted" to the primary level. Again, look carefully into your own heart to decide what *you want.*

The role (or plight, some might say) of the person in the position of secondary partner in polyamory requires some special flexibility and a willingness to yield (which is not the same as emotional submissiveness). As with polyamory itself, being a secondary is not for everyone.

My personal attitude, from experience being in the secondary role as well as the primary, is that I enjoy being a secondary (as well as a primary). Yes, sometimes I have had to shift or cancel plans to be with my secondary sweetie, and I have had the entire sexual relationship (but not the friendship) canceled or suspended by my secondary partner—once when my secondary was herself single but decided she wanted to seek someone for remarriage and thought (rightly, I think) that it would be simpler to find someone with the same goal if she were not sexually involved in a secondary relationship; another time when my secondary partner called a moratorium on the sexual aspects of her several secondary relationships in order to work on issues with her husband (again, rightly so).

My attitude is that I am delighted to have had those experiences with both those women (among other lovely secondary relationships over time).

Some people, though, find it personally troublesome not to be on an equal footing in a love relationship with another of their lover's partners (their lover's primary). There is nothing wrong with this attitude, and you will need to decide for yourself whether you find the experience of being in the secondary role to be a net positive, or not.

Keep in mind, if you are new to the secondary role, that being a secondary takes some getting used to, as can polyamory itself if your relationship experience to date has been of the mainstream monamorous variety.

The attitude of some people towards being a secondary also seems to be affected by whether they themselves are in a primary relationship (so that any secondary relationship would *feel* secondary to them as well as to their secondary partner), or whether they have no one else in their life but their secondary partner does have a primary. In the latter situation, the secondary partner without a primary may come to feel a desire to elevate the relationship to a higher (more "primary") level than circumstances allow, or may more acutely feel the negative side of having to yield plans and calendar slots to someone else.

Of course this is perfectly understandable, so, especially if you have no primary partner yourself, you may wish to keep these factors in mind if you have the opportunity to develop a new secondary relationship. Pay close attention to your emotional reactions to situations that bring your secondary status into sharp relief (reschedulings, cancellations, etc.), so you can decide if this relationship is a net positive or negative for you.

2.12. Sexual alphabet soup.

A number of sexual combinations are possible involving three or more people, depending on the sexual orientation of each and whether or not a given two people are sexually attracted to each other. What follows here applies equally to committed primary groups, to combinations of committed (primary) partners and secondary partners, or to more casual sexual get-togethers.

In a threesome (as noted in section 2.04), if all three people are hetero, there will be a sexual "V", meaning that the two people (A and B) who are of the same gender will be at the upper points of the "V", with the third person (C), of the other gender, at the angle of the "V". If all are together in the same bed, A and B can give C sexual pleasure simultaneously. C can give sexual pleasure to both A and B simultaneously, or C can be sexual with A or B, one at a time.

If the two people of the same gender are both bisexual, then a sexual triangle becomes possible. Since we often describe other sexual combinations with letters, we could name this by the Greek letter "delta", "Δ", but in practice this term is not often heard.

With four people, naturally more different combinations become possible. The four can pair off into two twosomes. There are four different threesome possibilities—or of course all four together.

There are two other possibilities with four. One arrangement could be called the "Z" (a "V" plus one more stroke), in which A shares sex with B, B with C, C with D, but no other pairings share sex together. The other possibility is the "Y", in which A (at the center of the "Y") shares sex with B, C, and D (at the extremities of the "Y"), but there is no sex in any other pairing.

With five people, if they have the same linear sexual arrangement, the "Z" expands to a "W". The "Y" could become an "X". And so on.

2.12

Of course as more and more people are added, the diagram of connections becomes quite entangled! If you draw a chart of a number of people as small circles with their interconnecting relationship lines snaking around, it starts to look amazingly much like a microscopic view of a brain, with neurons at intervals from each other that are connected with each other through synapses. What do you suppose we are evolving with these growing polyamorous groups?

~ 3 ~
Ethical Considerations

Contents:
3.01. Overview.
3.02. When your potential new lover is in a primary relationship.
3.03. A "cheater" as intermediary.
3.04. If your own primary relationship is weak or flawed.
3.05. Covering for the lies of others.
3.06. Appeals to protect a partner.
3.07. Other ethical dilemmas.
3.08. Keeping confidentialities and respecting privacy.
3.09. Requests for confidentiality.
3.10. Speaking up with nonpoly people.

♥ ♥ ♥

Once upon a time there was a small town, full of decent, neighborly folks.

This town was just big enough to support two churches, on opposite sides of town.

It happened that Rev. Al, who served the church on the east side of town, lived on the west side; and Rev. Bernie, who was the minister at the west-side church, lived on the east side. Both preachers liked to get back and forth by bicycle when the weather was nice. Each morning and each afternoon, as they passed each other in the center of town on their bikes, they'd give each other a friendly wave.

One morning as Rev. Al was pedaling toward his church, he saw his friend Bernie coming toward him—on foot. Al stopped and said, "Bernie! Why are you walking? Where's your bicycle?"

3

"I wish I knew!" said Bernie. "I have no idea! It just disappeared!"

"Disappeared?"

"Yeah! It's very strange. I hate to think that anyone in our town might be capable of such a thing, but the only possibility I can think of is that someone must have stolen my bicycle!" said Bernie.

"Oh, that's just awful!" said Al.

After a moment, Al's face lit up. "Say, I have an idea!" he said. "You know, nearly everyone in this town is a member either of your church or mine. This coming Sunday morning, let's both preach on the Ten Commandments, and when we get to 'Thou shalt not steal,' we bear down on it pretty hard. Odds are pretty good that whoever stole your bike will be in one or the other of our congregations, and maybe, when they hear that, they'll get a guilty conscience and return the bike."

"Yeah, I like that idea!" said Bernie. "Okay, let's try that!"

The following Monday morning, as Al was pedaling through town toward his office, he saw his friend Bernie coming toward him—and Bernie was back on his bicycle! As both preachers braked to a stop, Al said, "Bernie! You got your bike back! It looks like our plan worked!"

"Yes, it did," said Bernie, rather sheepishly. "But not the way we expected."

"How's that?"

"Well," said Bernie, "Yesterday morning, just as we agreed, I was giving my sermon on the Ten Commandments. But when I got down to 'Thou shalt not commit adultery,' I remembered where I left my bicycle!"

♥ ♥ ♥

3.01. Overview.

We noted at the very beginning of this book, in section 1.01, that one of the cornerstones of polyamory, distinguishing it from the mainstream sexual practice of "affairs", is ethical, respectful consideration of other people's feelings, including honesty, among other things—openly revealing your activities and feelings, especially to those closest in your life, but also to others with whom you have some involvement, sexual or otherwise. This openness and honesty is a basic essential in honoring one's commitment to keeping one's marriage or comparable committed relationship foremost in one's heart, giving it priority over other relationships that might develop.

A very high percentage of those in standard, mainstream marriages or relationships indulge in outside sexual "affairs" at one time or another, but they try to keep their affairs secret from their spouses or partners, with tragic consequences that are reflected in the separation and divorce rates, not to mention enormous psychological damage both to perpetrators, to their partners, and to any children in the home.

There is a more ethical, respectful way to treat people, a way that will improve life for all of us, polyamorous or not, adult or child—and I'm not referring here to the old advice simply to abstain from all but your primary sexual involvement. Polyamory doesn't demand that.

Basically, it does boil down to a matter of respect for others—which is also what the Golden Rule is about—and about keeping your primary relationship primary. Ask yourself if *you* would want to be lied to, or misled, or kept in the dark, especially by your primary. The way to get others to treat you straightforwardly is for this to be your own rigorous ongoing behavior toward others, especially your primary—even when this is difficult.

3.01

Physicists and spiritual leaders around the world agree on the principle of reciprocity, of which the Golden Rule is one wording; it's just that physicists and spiritual leaders word it differently.

Isaac Newton, one of the founders of modern physics in the 17th century, formulated this fundamental law of physics: "For every action there is an equal and opposite reaction."

The Buddha, more than two thousand years before Newton, taught us about karma—the same principle as it applies in the realm of human thoughts and deeds.

Going back probably a lot earlier than the Buddha, through the oral tradition, shamans and bodhisattvas and prophets and rabbis and messiahs and saints have been continually reminding us that if we treat others with respect and honesty, it will be returned to us. If not, then not. Our modern "street sense" expresses this as "what goes around comes around." It's still the same idea, the same fundamental wisdom.

Of course, there is the occasional "bad apple" who will take advantage of our good nature and mistreat us regardless of how well we treat them—but that is the narrow, short-term perspective, and the bad apples do not invalidate the general principle. What the bad apples do will "come around" to them too, sooner or later.

We need not belabor these basic truths, but it may be worthwhile to briefly restate this ancient wisdom here, because it does underlie all our ethical considerations of how to relate with those who are close to us, as well as with others.

But philosophers have noted for thousands of years that no matter how carefully we guide our actions by high ethical principles, we will sometimes run into an ethical dilemma, a gray area, where the best ethical choice between two courses of action is not at all obvious.

This chapter will suggest some ways to deal with ethical dilemmas in the realm of polyamorous relationships, such as whether to get involved with someone sexually who is in another relationship. Chapter 6 looks at communication techniques in other situations, and other relationship skills. Chapter 7 looks at resolving issues more generally, including balancing one partner's wishes and feelings against those of another, for example when you may want to compromise or yield and when you may feel that it is better not to, as well as how to clear your conscience about a past or present secret "affair", in the most empathetic way and the way most likely to keep your primary relationship intact and help it become even stronger.

3.02. When your potential new lover is in a primary relationship.

This section applies equally well whether you are in a primary relationship yourself or you are unattached.

Let's say you become interested in someone who is already in a primary relationship. Your new love interest is willing to share sex with you, but they tell you not to let their spouse or partner know—or they may imply the secrecy indirectly by saying something like, "I'll have to call you; please don't call me, because my husband might answer the phone." Or, "Please call me only at work."

Would it be an "affair" or something else? If you are asked not to contact your new interest at home and the like, that strongly suggests that they are willing to start a secret "affair" with you—but there are a couple of other possibilities. One is that your potential new lover may have thoroughly discussed the question of secondary relationships with their primary partner and they have come to a "don't ask, don't tell" agreement. In such an arrangement, the two primary partners agree that each may develop secondary relationships, but they *choose* not to know anything specific as to whether such a relationship actually exists, who the hypothetical secondary partner is, when they get together, etc.

You can see the stark difference between not knowing because you *don't want* to know, and not knowing because your primary is lying to you. Therein lies the ethical crux of the matter. (See sections 2.03 and 2.04 for further discussion about "don't ask, don't tell" and other varieties of agreement possible between primary partners.)

There is at least one more possibility about the situation in your new interest's home, if they ask you to keep your involvement with them secret. (We warned you that polyamory is complex!) Your love interest may be in a marriage or cohabiting partnership that is emotionally dead or nearly so, but the two people continue under the same roof for economic reasons, because of the children, or just lack of initiative by either of them to move out. In this situation, even if they had an explicit vow or agreement of monamory early on, they each may consider that agreement effectively as dead as the relationship now, so that neither of them really cares what their nominally primary partner does with others. Their own sex life may not exist at this point.

Here's another real-life ethical dilemma known to the author. Person A (a woman) and B are married, and both want to preserve the marriage. A has a strong libido, but her husband, B, has little or no interest in sex, not with A and not with anyone else. But B is unwilling to allow A the freedom for seeking sexual fulfillment with others (a poly/mono relationship—see section 2.08—but with little or no sex in the primary relationship).

A's choice is either to pursue her sexual fulfillment in one or more outside affairs secretly, which relieves the temptation to leave the marriage over the issue of the sexual imbalance, but involves lying to her husband; or to refrain from the outside sexual involvements, which allows A to be truthful with her husband but places great stress on the marriage because of A's sexual frustration.

If *you* have the opportunity to be a lover for A in that situation (as I did), would you accept, considering that you are doing your part to preserve the stability of A's marriage? Or would you decline, on grounds of not being an accomplice to A's deceitfulness, even though that would mean further threatening A's marriage? (Don't get hung up over your own gender and orientation here; if necessary, imagine that A is male.)

We'll get back in a moment to the question of whether a possible new secondary relationship would be a secret affair or "don't ask, don't tell"—but does it even matter to you which is the case?

Should this concern you? You could take the position that if your new love interest is willing to engage in behavior that could be destructive to their home relationship (if it *is* a secret "affair" that's being offered to you), that is their concern and not yours. You are not their parent, and you are both competent adults. Many polyamorists follow this policy. I personally feel there is more to this situation, however, which you as the would-be secondary would be wise to consider.

At the beginning of this chapter, in section 3.01, we noted the universal law of reciprocity, which applies just as much in human interactions as in the interactions of billiard balls or worlds according to the laws of physics. "What goes around comes around."

If you engage in a sexual involvement with someone who is in a primary relationship, and your involvement constitutes an "affair" for your lover in violation of your lover's vows or relationship agreement with their primary, then, although your lover would certainly be the main culprit in their primary's eyes, you are at least an accomplice. You are creating a negative karmic connection between yourself, your lover, and your lover's primary.

3.02

If you choose to ignore these metaphysical concerns, there is still the fact, very much in this physical world, that by sharing sex with this new interest of yours, you will be contributing somehow or other to rocking the boat for your lover *and* their primary. (We are leaving aside for the moment the situation described above, in which A has a strong sex drive, B does not and refuses to allow A to seek satisfaction elsewhere.) How does this fit with your basic sense of fairness and decency toward other people in general? How would you like it if *you* were treated that way?

Another concern very much in this world is whether you can trust what your new would-be lover says to you. You have already learned that they are willing to lie to or withhold basic information from their primary. Can you be sure you are hearing the truth when, for example, they tell you that they have been tested free of STDs?

Let's suppose you decide to share sex with this person *only* if you can be reasonably sure that doing so would *not* violate any agreement, vow, or assumption between them and their primary. Now it *is* relevant for you to find out which of the three possibilities described above is the case.

First, find out the details. The first thing you may want to do is to ask your new love interest whether the situation would be a secret "affair", a case of "don't ask, don't tell", or an involvement that wouldn't matter to your interest's primary because that supposedly "primary" relationship is really emotionally dead.

The best time to make this inquiry could be right after your interest asks you to keep your involvement just between you, asks you not to call, etc. When your interest tells you something like that, it easily leads to your asking the reason for the request for secrecy.

If an "affair". If the answer is that the reason for secrecy is because your interest's primary assumes there are no outside sexual involvements, and would be upset to learn of one, then you know you would be incurring that karmic debt and/or treating the primary unfairly, as discussed above. You also know now that your new interest cannot be trusted always to tell the truth. If you have resolved in yourself not to allow yourself to get into such secret involvements, then you may feel that the matter is now decided: You have to tell your new interest, "Sorry, I'd like to take you to bed, but not under these circumstances."

Or, if confronted with the situation of A and B above with their unbalanced libidos, you may decide to make an exception to your general principle and accept involvement with A, thereby helping A stay content at home, even though you and A would then have to maintain secrecy the same as for any "affair".

If "don't ask, don't tell". If your interest tells you that they and their primary have agreed to polyamory but have further agreed not to volunteer any further information nor ask each other for it ("don't ask, don't tell"), then you may conclude that you are ethically free to proceed—if you trust enough that this person is telling you the truth. See section 6.13, and below in this section, for more about trust.

At some point, though (it doesn't have to be immediately), you *may* want to draw your lover into a conversation about the disadvantages of the "don't ask, don't tell" policy, simply as a friend seeking to help your lover and their primary find the best form of relating openly. This is discussed in more detail in section 2.03.

If a dead primary relationship. If your new interest's nominally primary partner evidently does not really care if your interest shares sex with anyone else, because the relationship is emotionally dead, then again you may conclude that you are ethically free to proceed (again, if you trust what you are being told), since you will not be going against any *active* vows or expectations. In the case of a dead primary relationship, it is reasonable not to trouble one's nominal primary with knowledge about other emotional or sexual involvements that they would not care about, and so it is also reasonable to ask you, a new secondary, not to phone the home or do other things that would reveal your secondary relationship.

Taking their word for it. We've noted above that if someone shows a willingness to lie to and hide information from their own primary partner, then you lose some of your own trust in their veracity. And yet, if you decide to go ahead with a sexual involvement with this person, then you probably have no choice but to accept their word for certain things, such as a claim that they have a "don't ask, don't tell" agreement with their primary (you can't verify with the other primary without violating the "don't tell" part), or a claim that their primary relationship is emotionally dead.

If you happen to be acquainted with your potential secondary's primary, you might be able to draw that person into a conversation about the *general* topic of varieties of relationship arrangements, while carefully avoiding revealing your own interest in their partner. You might hear a comment affirming that they have a "don't ask, don't tell" arrangement—or you might hear something like, "Polyamory? Definitely not! My wife/husband and I have vowed not to get involved sexually with anyone else." Now you have the information you were looking for. You've been lied to.

About your only other recourse for verification, if you have mutual acquaintances, is to ask someone else their opinion of the person's veracity. Then again, as pointed out in section 6.13, in order to live a personally fulfilling life we must sometimes be willing to trust others even when we have less than perfect evidence as to whether the person is trustworthy or not. This may be one of those times.

In this sort of uncertain situation, when you are not sure how trustworthy your new love interest is but you have taken all reasonable steps to ascertain the truth, at least you can take comfort in the knowledge that if they *are* lying to you about their home situation, the responsibility for any negative consequences is entirely theirs, not shared by you. You've done what you could.

3.03. A "cheater" as intermediary.

Like the case described in section 3.02, reasonable people could decide this one differently. I'm presenting this possible scenario here as another illustration that ethics does have gray areas. You can think about how *you* would react with the hypothetical situation described in this section.

Genders don't really matter here, but to help you keep the cast of characters here straight, I'll assign genders and arbitrarily use the beginning of the alphabet to name women, the end of the alphabet for men. You might find it helpful to draw a chart of the relationships involved here. (Sometimes a chart can be helpful in real-life polyamory as well!)

Let's suppose that a fellow whom we'll call Z lives with a woman, A. Z lets another woman, B, know that he would like to start a secondary relationship. B is initially interested, so the two of them chat some, to get acquainted. Z mentions to B that he lives with A, and that he also has an intimate relationship going with another woman, C, who has no committed relationship and lives alone.

Z honestly reveals to B that the woman he lives with, A, does not know about his sexual involvement with C. Z tells B that although he and A are deeply committed and have an understanding that they will be sexually exclusive (monamorous), Z says that he personally feels a strong need for more sexual variety, a need that A does not understand or accept; and so his relationship with C is clandestine. Z also would not tell A about B, if B agreed to become involved with Z.

3.03

Because this secrecy in a committed relationship would violate B's own ethical standards (as described in section 3.02), B tells Z, after she has learned these facts, that she is not willing to share sexual intimacy with him, even though she finds him attractive.

This much is fairly straightforward. If I were in B's place there, I would make the same decision.

Meanwhile, however, before B decides not to go further with Z, Z also has some online chats with B's primary partner, Y. (B, being open and honest with Y, has informed Y of her own earlier chats with Z and her growing interest in Z.) Z mentions to Y that another single female friend, D, might be interested in meeting with both Z and Y, maybe for a sexual threesome if everyone "clicks". This might happen whether or not B decides to participate. Let's stipulate here also that Z and Y are hetero, and so it would have been a sexual "V", with Z and Y connecting sexually with D, but with no sex between Z and Y.

D and Y do become introduced in person, and they "click", and they became sexually attracted to each other.

Now we get to the question. Would it violate ethical principles for Y to become involved in a sexual threesome with Z and D? (In case your head is spinning by now with all the interconnections, let's remember that Z has revealed that he's conducting an affair with one woman, C, in secret from his primary, and so an involvement with any other women would also be in secret. Since the two men, Z and Y, are both hetero, Y would be sexually involved only with D, not with Z, in a Z-D-Y threesome.) What if Y and D become sexual without Z present?

What would you do in Y's place? If you want to think about it a while, stop reading for now, because I'll give my take on this in the next paragraph.

If I were Y, I would feel that such a sexual threesome would *not violate* my ethics, since I would share sex only with D, who herself would not be "cheating" on anyone, since she had no committed relationship. So, if the opportunity had arisen and if she and I had both been interested, I would have proceeded. Of course, my knowledge that D was an accomplice to Z's cheating on A might lower my estimation of her in my own eyes, maybe to the point that I wouldn't be interested in sharing sex with her. But that's a separate question. D might have other positive qualities that (in my mind) would outweigh our disagreement about that ethical question.

I would apply the same considerations if D were interested in sharing sex with me separately (if I were Y), not including Z.

Again, this is just how *I* would decide that hypothetical question, and you may look at the same facts and come to a different conclusion. Once again, ethics is full of interesting gray areas!

3.04. *If your own primary relationship is weak or flawed.*

This book stresses the importance of complete openness and honesty with your primary partner(s), and the importance of working to bolster your own home relationship. But another fundamental truth of life is that there are no fundamental truths! Things aren't black or white, as section 3.03 suggests. Life is messy, full of ambiguities and contradictions. (Let's be honest—it would be boring if it weren't.)

Openness and honesty certainly is *one of the most important* principles in poly life, or indeed in life by any paradigm. But so is personal integrity. What if these conflict?

Suppose you are in a marriage or committed relationship with the traditional mutual commitment of sexual exclusivity which the two of you made to each other early on, probably while you were both in the throes of NRE. After some time you decide you would like to open up the relationship and adopt a polyamorous agreement with your partner.

3.04

You may have come to the realization that you are really polyamorous by *orientation,* not just lifestyle choice (see section 1.04).

The two of you discuss it, but let's suppose that even after discussion your partner does not wish to adopt polyamory and adamantly resists the notion of allowing you to have secondary sexual relationships on your own (a poly/mono relationship, as described in section 2.08). You seek professional counseling together, but this also fails to bring the two of you to a workable consensus. Where does that leave you, individually?

If your relationship is solid, then your only ethical choice appears to be to continue to adhere to the agreement to exclusivity that the two of you made earlier. But section 3.02 points out that a committed relationship can fade or deteriorate, for whatever reasons, even though the couple continue to live together, so that the external appearance no longer reflects the reality between the two people involved. They are no longer focusing their energies fully or primarily on that relationship, and no amount of further mutual effort is likely to resurrect the former degree of connectedness between them. Another possibility is that although the relationship remains strong in other respects, the two partners come upon an issue that they are unable to resolve and that is fundamental to the basic personality needs of one or both of them.

Section 3.02 approached the situation of a deteriorating primary relationship from the perspective of someone outside that relationship—from the perspective of a potential new *secondary* partner of one of them. This section looks at that situation, and the situation of the fundamental impasse, with the assumption that you are one of the *primary* partners.

We are also assuming here that at this point the two of you *have* already discussed the issue at length in good faith, and also that you have sought professional counseling, all to no avail; or that you have repeatedly *asked* your partner to discuss and seek counseling, but your partner will not cooperate. This was already mentioned earlier in this section, but it needs to be stressed, because you would be stepping out onto ethical thin ice to enter into another sexual relationship without your partner's knowledge or agreement, and then to try to justify to yourself keeping that secret from your primary partner on grounds that you and your primary "just have that basic irreconcilable difference", if you have *not* taken those measures to reach some consensus, or made a good-faith attempt. Be honest with yourself.

You may feel that you can justify keeping knowledge of an outside sexual involvement from your primary partner if you have concluded either that your primary relationship has deteriorated to the point that your initial commitment of exclusivity is no longer binding, with no reasonable chance of rebuilding; or else that your primary's unmoving position over some time forces you into the position that your basic nature (orientation) just requires you to take action on your own, even if you are trying to maintain your primary relationship as strong and healthy as you can in other respects, in spite of all the well-known risks and consequences of taking action without your partner's knowledge. In other words, the situation is such that you cannot both honor your partner's wishes and also be true to your own basic nature.

Of course only you can judge whether this is your situation. This step cannot be taken lightly. Be honest with yourself (as I said), and don't be hasty—but also be true to yourself. Be careful not to confuse "I want that a lot" with "That's my basic nature."

3.05. *Covering for the lies of others.*

Sometimes you may learn or suspect that someone (A) has lied to their primary (B). If then you are speaking with B, is it ethically better to cover for the lie, or to speak the truth frankly as best you know it? Maybe A has asked you to cover for them, maybe not.

3.05

An example of this is described in section 1.08, in the situation in which you are interested in developing a secondary relationship with A, who claims to have a "don't ask, don't tell" relationship with their partner (B); in order to test whether A is telling you the truth, you engage B in a general conversation about polyamory without revealing your interest in A; and B tells you that (contrary to what A told you) A and B do not practice any form of polyamory, but are have a sexually exclusive relationship.

Suppose B then comes back with something like, "How did you get the idea that my husband/wife and I are sexually open?" How do you respond to this? You could attempt to cover A's lie by improvising a "white lie" of your own, stating that evidently you were somehow confused; you misheard; you were thinking of someone else; etc. Or you can state frankly that A told you that they had a "don't ask, don't tell" relationship with B—which reveals to B that A has lied to him or her.

I personally favor telling B the truth, for practical reasons as well as ethics. As is well known, anyone who tells a lie starts a chain-reaction need for further lies, to cover the first one. ("Oh, what a tangled web we weave When first we practise to deceive!"—Sir Walter Scott, in "Marmion".) This can expand out to include others who may be willing to participate in the deceit. In the conversation here between you and B, if you invent some cover-up story in talking with B in order to protect A, now you are also drawn into the "tangled web", no matter how innocent your "white lie" may seem.

From an ethical standpoint, there is no moral obligation for one person to help someone else maintain deceits. If I were in that situation, I'd speak the truth to B—gently but directly. If B then confronted A, A's stew would be of their own making.

3.06. Appeals to protect a partner.

A female poly friend of mine (A) told me of an instance in which a man who claimed to be poly (B) wanted to start a sexual relationship with her, but B told her that his primary partner (C) would have her feelings hurt if she found out that he was involved with A, and so B asked A not to let it get back to C for that reason.

A agreed to this, initially—but when C did find out, some months later, there was the usual great storm and feelings of betrayal of C by B, the typical reaction when anyone learns that their committed partner has indulged in a secret affair.

With "20/20 hindsight" (as A acknowledged to me), it seems rather obvious that A should not have taken B at his word about the reasons for wanting secrecy. A came out of that unpleasant experience with the sense of "a life lesson learned".

3.07. Other ethical dilemmas.

Sometimes an ethical dilemma seems frustratingly resistant to sorting it out and deciding one way or the other. Here is an example, another real situation that I learned about. This case is one of those convoluted poly situations involving several parties. As I did in section 3.03, I will use the end of the alphabet for males, the beginning of the alphabet for females. And, again, you might be able to keep track of the various connections better by drawing a chart.

Persons Z and A are a married couple. Z has a secondary relationship with another woman, B, who in turn has a secondary relationship with a man, Y.

C is a woman who has a friendship with both A and B. In a conversation between A and C, A confides to C that A "suspects that Z is having an affair." (Presumably this "affair" is the relationship between Z and B.) C later describes this conversation to B, who tells Y.

3.07

A's choice of words, that Z might be "having an affair," strongly suggested to C (and later to B and Y, when they heard the story) that A believed that her relationship with Z was monamorous; it follows that if Z and A do have this commitment to exclusivity, then Z has lied to B in claiming that he has a polyamorous relationship with A.

Where does this put B with regard to Z? Does B, C, or Y have a moral obligation to speak to A about Z's sexual involvement with B and the apparently different story that Z has told B about whether he has a polyamorous relationship with A? Now that B strongly suspects that Z has been lying to her, should she break off her sexual involvement with Z, or confront Z to see if he can clarify the situation or defend himself?

You may wish to ponder this situation yourself for a bit before reading further. As often happens, there is no single right answer to this one. In fact I do not know what the parties involved finally decided, but this situation was presented to a poly email discussion list (by Y), which is how I learned of it, and in the next paragraph I will describe the consensus of advice offered by several subscribers to that list.

The general consensus of several people who responded to Y's posting to the list was that someone (B, C, or Y)—and probably B would be in the best position to do so—should approach Z and let him know that stories are going around that he has told different things to A and to B, with the strong suggestion that he has concealed from his wife, A, the existence of his relationship with B. Give Z the opportunity to come clean to A himself (perhaps along the model described in sections 7.06 through 7.08). If Z is cheating on A (as it appears to us on the outside), then the emotional impact on A is likely to be less intense and potentially more positive if A learns of the situation directly from Z than if she hears of it from B, C, or Y. The prospects will be much better for Z and A to heal this broken piece in their relationship if Z is the one who talks to A.

As a sort of footnote, if this situation is what it appears to be—that Z has falsely promised exclusivity to A while falsely telling B that he and A are polyamorous so that he can carry on a sexual involvement with B—the situation illustrates the importance of verifying assertions whenever possible before becoming sexually involved with someone who is in a committed relationship. When Z and B first became interested in each other as potential sexual partners, if B had asked to meet A and talk with her (see section 3.02), and maybe by talking with the mutual friend C, she *might* have either gleaned useful information from Z or else might have had suspicions aroused depending on how Z answered or on what C told her about the Z-A relationship.

3.08. Keeping confidentialities and respecting privacy.

People in the mainstream are well trained not to speak freely about certain topics, including sex. We in the polyamory community have had to work against this social conditioning in some ways in order to maintain solidly open communication habits among primary partners and others.

This openness and completeness of communication is so thoroughly accepted in the polyamory community (and rightly so) that we sometimes need to remind ourselves of the other side of the coin—the right and expectation of *privacy* by others, including other poly people with whom we may be intimately involved. If I am chatting casually with a friend of mine, it is too easy to say something like, "My wife is starting a new relationship with Bob in our poly discussion group. Bob was over at our place last Saturday, and wow, you should've heard him yell when he came!"

When we think about it, we immediately realize that this comment inappropriately invades the privacy of both people involved, the wife and her secondary—unless we *happen* to know that *both* are comfortable with sharing this sort of juicy tidbit with the other person that we are speaking with—and, for that matter, even sharing the fact that they have become lovers.

Everyone has different feelings about how private they wish to keep this part of their life, even among other polyamorous people who may be friends of all concerned or who are presumably sympathetic at least to the existence of the various intertwined relationships. It is best, then, not to reveal either the existence of a secondary relationship or (even more so) details of sexual behavior as in the above example, unless we know that all parties are comfortable with the disclosure. If in doubt, keep it private.

You can often protect privacy by not naming names, of course, but if you do that when talking with someone who is part of a fairly small group of acquaintances and friends (as is typical of local polyamory groups), also be careful not to reveal enough other details about a person or situation that a good inference of identity can be made.

3.09. *Requests for confidentiality.*

Sometimes someone will ask us to keep some personal information that they tell us private or confidential. Sometimes this request comes before we've been given the information, sometimes after.

If someone asks you to keep confidential something that they have not yet told you, then you have the freedom to decide whether you want to honor that request, for whatever reason. Maybe you feel it would violate your ethical principles to keep the information completely confidential (even from your own primary); maybe you simply don't trust your own memory enough to be sure that you'll remember not to blurt out this information. In this case, if you respond, "Sorry, I can't promise never to pass on whatever you want to tell me," or "Well, my primary and I have no secrets between us, but I could agree to keep it confidential from everyone else," then the other person can choose whether to tell you whatever it is.

Sometimes the other person will tell you something first, and *then* will ask you, "Please don't tell anyone else," or "Please don't tell your primary," or some other specific person. You are under no moral obligation to honor this request, since the information was given to you before you had the opportunity to decline the request for confidentiality. You can honor it or not, totally or selectively. For example, keeping the secret from your primary may violate your overriding agreement for complete openness and honesty with your primary, but you may decide that you can agree after the fact to refrain from telling anyone else.

3.10. *Speaking up with nonpoly people.*

Polyamory is steadily becoming more widely known in society at large, but *acceptance* by nonpoly people can be a lot slower to come than mere *awareness,* as has been the case earlier with homosexuals and other groups—different groups in different cultures. Thus, we may still occasionally hear remarks that criticize polyamory or polyamorous people, or just show a lack of understanding.

An example of this might be, "Ann is so loose! I've heard that she has five boyfriends, in addition to living with another guy!" Or, "John is so insensitive toward his wife! The other day I saw him holding hands with another woman and kissing her, right out on the sidewalk in their neighborhood where people who know him and his wife might see them!"

How do you respond when you hear remarks of this sort? Do you just give a weak smile and a shrug and change the subject? Do you try to enlighten the person making these remarks? Do you indignantly put your hands on your hips and give the speaker a lecture about bigotry against those with a different lifestyle?

3.10

The hands-on-hips option was not a serious suggestion. I cannot envision any situation in which the scolding technique would be effective. It is simply counterproductive, because it casts you in the role of ersatz parent, the other person in the role of child, and no one will be willing to listen or engage in dialog under those circumstances. You'll be dismissed as a kook.

Try to enlighten when possible. Because of the need to educate mainstream society about polyamory and polyamorists (a solidly ethical need), I strongly favor attempting to enlighten the person who makes this sort of unaware remark, when circumstances permit a brief comment in response. Society at large can indeed become enlightened in this way, one brief conversation at a time. It has worked before, with other misunderstood or marginalized groups.

Of course circumstances do not always permit, as with a remark from a stranger overheard in an elevator. But even in that situation, before one of you exits the elevator, you might at least be able to toss off a quick remark to the other person, maybe along the lines of, "Well, different people have different ways of relating ethically with each other."

What to say. You do not need to go into a long sermon about the philosophy and ethics underlying polyamory, the varieties, and so on—unless you both have plenty of time and the other person shows genuine interest in learning about polyamory in some detail. In this sort of situation it is enough just to say something brief that focuses on the fact that different people openly choose different ways of living and loving, and as long as no one is being deceived or hurt, there is nothing wrong with their choices. You can elaborate if and to the extent that circumstances permit and the other person is interested, maybe briefly describing your own particular variety of poly living.

In the example above about "Ann" who was alleged to have a live-in partner and five other boyfriends, you could say something like, "Well, I don't know the particulars about Ann, but some people are comfortable with multiple relationships. What matters is whether someone *knows* that their live-in partner has other lovers. Open and honest communication is the key. If someone is okay with their partner having other lovers, there's no problem. If one of them is keeping *secrets* from the other, then there's a problem."

Be careful of the closet. "Ann" and "John" in the above examples are *probably* out of the closet, if they let their polyamory be so publicly seen and known—but that should never be assumed. If you know for a fact that someone is totally open about their polyamory, fine. Otherwise, it is ethically best to protect their privacy with phrases such as I used above, "I don't know the particulars about Ann, but some people…." Notice what this phrasing does. It removes the commentary from being about Ann specifically—you are not confirming or denying that she is polyamorous, or that she has many lovers. It makes your statement generic, commenting about "some people". See Chapter 9 about the closet.

~ 4 ~

Sexual Hygiene

Contents:
4.01. Overview.
4.02. Agreement with your primary partner(s).
4.03. Discuss with potential new sex partners.
4.04. Genital safe sex practices.
4.05. Oral safe sex practices.
4.06. Anal safe sex practices.
4.07. Dildos, vibrators, and other sex toys.
4.08. Starting condom use after going condomless for a while.
4.09. Getting tested.
4.10. The incubation period.
4.11. Criteria for fluid-bondedness.
4.12. Making safe sex more fun.
4.13. Using condoms among primaries or other fluid-bonded partners.
4.14. List of STDs.

♥ ♥ ♥

Why does it take ten million sperm to fertilize one egg?
Because none of them will stop to ask for directions.

♥ ♥ ♥

4.01. Overview.

What is an STD? The acronym stands for "sexually transmitted disease". It's also sometimes called a "sexually transmitted infection",

4.01

STI. As the name suggests, an STD is any disease caused by a microbe (a bacterium, a virus, or a parasite) that can pass from one person's body to another during any sort of sexual contact, such as genital-genital, oral-genital, or genital-anal.

Some STDs can also be transmitted in nonsexual ways, for example when a drug addict uses a syringe previously used by an infected person, when a tattooist or body piercer uses a contaminated needle, from mother to baby before or during childbirth, when breast-feeding, by transfusion of contaminated blood, when the blood or other bodily fluid of one person accidentally enters a skin break on another person, by casually touching an open sore or other skin break and then touching someone else on a spot where the microbe can enter the body—and in one case (trichomoniasis) just by sharing a damp towel.

This chapter is concerned only with disease transmission through some form of sexual contact, and with diseases that can be transmitted that way (that is, STDs), although nonsexual methods by which STDs can also be transmitted are also mentioned.

Balance risk and benefit. Anyone who even occasionally enjoys sexual involvement other than with their primary partner(s) in an exclusive relationship incurs some risk of contracting an STD. Even the "safe" sex practices discussed in this chapter are not 100% safe; they just reduce the risk substantially. For this reason many people prefer to use the phrase "safer sex" rather than "safe sex". I'll say "safe sex", but keep in mind that as long as you are sexually active (with the exception of monamory or polyfidelity), you incur *some* risk.

The only 100% safe "sex" practice is no sex—refrain. This should certainly be one of your options that you consider when you weigh how much risk you would be incurring (for yourself and for your fluid-bonded partner(s)) in sharing sex with a potential new partner.

4.01

Each individual must decide how much risk they are willing to accept and how cautious they want to be. When two or more people are fluid-bonded, they need to discuss this question together (concerning other partners for either of them) and come to a shared agreement. This agreement should become part of their relationship agreement. (See section 4.02 and Chapter 5).

After you read this chapter, especially the last section, section 4.14, recounting all the "bad news" about STDs, you may be tempted to renounce society altogether and join a Tibetan monastery. But the existence of STDs does not need to deter people altogether from enjoying sex with a variety of partners—after wisely choosing who those partners are, then cautiously following safe sex practices. Everything in life has risks; life involves balancing risks with benefits (and pleasure certainly counts as a benefit). If we try to hide in a cave against all risks—well, the cave might collapse on us.

The odds of being squashed by a collapsing cave are probably less than the risk of being hit by a car when bicycling on a road, or just walking across a city street (even when the sign says "Walk"). The decision for every road bicycling enthusiast (that includes your humble author), after donning brightly colored clothing and a helmet, installing reflectors and a mirror on the bicycle, and activating one's best common sense about what roads to ride on, is whether the residual risk is an acceptable "price" for the enjoyment and health benefits of regular bicycling.

We all take reasonable precautions against known risks, and then we go ahead with whatever level of risk remains. When we sit down in a car, we buckle our seat belt. When we slide into bed with anyone we are not reasonably sure of, we unwrap a condom.

Knowing that condoms do not reduce the risk of infection to zero, we are also careful about who we slide into bed with, and we also have ourselves tested at regular intervals. (See section 4.09.) So read this chapter, but don't be intimidated by it. If you're going to screw around, you need to know this stuff, at least in general terms.

If you become infected, or you suspect it. Needless to say, promptly see a health care provider—and immediately inform all your current sex partners, fluid-bonded or not. Also inform any potential new partners before testing (and retesting after the incubation period) confirms your state of health. If you are diagnosed with an STD, again inform any current or potential new partners, including those with whom you would use condoms, unless or until you are cured of it.

4.02. Agreement with your primary partner(s).

There is considerable room for personal preference in how you and your primary partner(s) decide to conduct your sex life with each other and with others—but it is important for you to come to some sort of agreement on the particulars. This should become part of your relationship agreement (see Chapter 5). If you do not have such an agreement in place, you might do something with someone else that you consider safe enough, but that your partner considers unacceptably risky—or vice versa. The resulting argument can be avoided by discussing these questions and reaching agreement in advance.

Here are the most basic questions to consider. You may think of others. I offer my own views on these questions, but, again, there is room for varying preferences with most of these.

    a. *When one of you shares sex with anyone else, will you use a condom?* I feel that condom use should at least be your "default" assumption, absent agreement otherwise among all who are fluid-bonded. That is, you and your fluid-bonded partner(s) may decide that a particular secondary is safe enough, because of

4.02

testing and their behavior practices, that you can go condomless with them. See section 4.11 for further discussion.

b. *Will condom use with others be an absolute requirement, or will you consider individual cases in which a particular secondary partner might be safe enough that you may become fluid-bonded with that person?* I feel that flexibility on condom use with others is good, with careful discussion as described below in (c) and in section 4.11.

c. *If you and your primary do consider becoming fluid-bonded with particular secondaries, what will be your criteria?* Asking the other person about recent testing is good, if you also ask them about possibly risky behavior (that is, condomless sex) or accidents (a condom slipping or breaking) during the six months prior to testing (the incubation period) and between testing and now. (See section 4.10.) If they have recently tested negative, and if there was no intentional or accidental skin-to-skin exposure during those times before and after, you and your primary or primaries may consider that sufficient for fluid-bondedness. If they have not recently been tested, I would want to see that done, with "clean" results, before agreeing to fluid-bondedness. Just saying something like "I've never been with anyone but my husband/wife since I was married" or "I haven't done any sexual playing around since college," etc., is not good enough, because (a) the spouse might have picked something up, then given it to this person; (b) this person might have picked something up, even years ago; (c) some people contract an STD in the womb, during birth, or in infancy from mother's milk, or from other nonsexual causes. Once infected, especially with viral STDs, the infections generally never go away, although they may remain symptomless. Claiming "I've never had any symptoms of anything" is meaningless, since a person infected with some diseases can go indefinitely with no symptoms. Testing is easy; it is commonly offered free by city and county health departments; and your new potential partner should want to be tested anyway for their own sake. Also see section 4.11.

d. *May one of you decide unilaterally, on the spot (for example, while out on a date with someone), that a new partner is safe enough for condomless sex, or must this be decided by both or all those fluid-bonded?* Generally I feel that this should be a shared decision, but a primary couple or fluid-bonded group might come up with explicit criteria which, if met, are enough without requiring further discussion among the fluid-bonded ones. For example, a fluid-bonded couple or group might agree that if the new person meets the criteria described in (c) above and in section 4.11, then one of their group may decide unilaterally (while out on a date with that person etc.) to proceed without condoms, not having to consult first with the other primary partner(s).

e. *How cautious do you want to be about oral sex?* Many people consider oral sex to be less risky than genital sex. This may be so, but there is still risk, more so with some kinds of oral sex. See the more complete discussion of this question in section 4.05 and the listing of specific STDs, with methods of transmission of each, in section 4.14.

f. *Will you allow anal penetration (if any of you desire it)?* Anal sex is somewhat more risky than vaginal sex because there are more bacteria and viruses in the rectum. For this reason, condomless anal sex is especially risky. This is discussed further in section 4.06.

g. *Will you allow vaginal sex with a female secondary who is menstruating?* I see no reason to preclude this normally, although the sexual partner of the menstruating woman should be careful that they have no skin breaks, even tiny ones such as a pimple or scratch, around their pubic area or on fingers used for play. The additional risk here is one-directional, from the menstruating woman to her sexual partner. If any doubt, refrain.

h. *What will you do if there is an accidental exposure, such as a condom that breaks or slips off?* At a minimum, the fluid-bonded partner who had something of this sort occur with a secondary should promptly inform the other fluid-bonded partner(s), who will then discuss together how to respond. Response probably should be kept flexible, depending on the particular circumstances—the degree of risk that may have occurred. At one extreme, the fluid-bonded partners could decide to do nothing, if the risk is small. At the other extreme, they might decide to use condoms themselves until the incubation period lapses and all parties then test clean. (If the risk is this great, hindsight might question the wisdom of having shared sex with that secondary partner even using condoms.)

4.03. Discuss with potential new sex partners.

When you are on a date with a new love interest, and as passion grows and the hormones are flowing in both of you, it can be difficult to call a pause long enough to exchange information about your respective states of health etc. Unless you just met each other five minutes ago at a swingers' party, hopefully each of you has already gotten some idea previously about the other's state of health and their habitual behaviors as you have made a start on getting to know each other but before the hormones start flowing.

It is an especially bad idea to be heading toward your first sexual encounter with someone new if either or both of you have been drinking or using any other mind-altering drug, since alcohol or the other drugs can impair the ability of your cerebrum to have this discussion and make the right decision, when your limbic brain and your hormones are shouting, *"I don't care about germs! I just wanna fuck! Now!"*

Regardless of how much of your new interest's state of health you have been able to learn before now, as the moment of your first sexual connection approaches, common sense would have you steer the conversation to the general topic of sexual health, hopefully before you start to get playful (it's easier not to start the groping than to back off half-way through).

You can work this into the conversation along with asking your new friend what sorts of sexual fun they prefer. What sorts of positions do you like? Do you like caresses on some parts of your body more than others? Any ticklish spots? Do you always use a condom with others? Have you ever experienced having two people giving you sexual pleasure at once? Does a gang-bang interest you? Do you enjoy sex parties? Do you enjoy sharing sex with people that you've just recently met? How much do you usually ask new partners about *their* sexual health?

Of course you would not want to make it seem like an interrogation, but you can weave carefully chosen questions such as these examples into a conversation to help you decide if this person is a reasonably good or poor health risk for you, even with condoms.

4.04. *Genital safe sex practices.*

Condoms. Condoms provide good protection against bacterial and viral STDs (as well as good contraceptive protection), but the protection is not 100%. A condom can break or slip off. Bodily fluids (especially menstrual blood, if a woman is flowing heavily) may get up above the top (open end) of the condom, so there is additional risk if a man has lesions (skin breaks) anywhere where that blood or other fluid can reach. If either partner has lesions around the pubic or groin area, not covered by the condom, or around the mouth where they kiss, this can sometimes be a route for STD infection.

Condoms come in a variety of sizes, reflecting the different lengths and thicknesses of penises. Condoms are also available with various bumps, ribbing, etc., on the outside, designed to give the receiver additional pleasure. For the man's (giver's) comfort a condom should not be too tight, but it should fit snugly so that it cannot easily be pulled off of a dry erect penis by tugging on the tip of it. If you are male and you are new to using condoms, you might want to try different sizes and kinds when alone to see which ones you like and which size fits best. Just be sure they aren't too loose.

For those allergic to latex (rubber), polyurethane (plastic) condoms are available.

Condoms should be stored away from excessive heat or cold. This means that a wallet and especially a car dash box are not good places to keep them. A purse or waistpack can be good storage, if the purse or waistpack is not itself left for any length of time in extreme heat or cold. Otherwise, store your condoms at home and take out a few when you think you might need them elsewhere on a date; put them in your pants pocket, purse, etc.

A woman should not assume that her male dating partner will have condoms available. Condoms are a shared responsibility. Whatever your gender, if you make sure you have condoms with you as you head out on a date, then you will not be in a dilemma if your dating partner did not bring any.

It's a good idea to have several condoms available, not just one, since problems can arise with a condom. For example, if the man is not quite hard enough, the condom may not go on readily, but it may become unrolled in the attempt. Then it cannot be used. Or it may slip off during sex. Again in that case, you need a new one. The one wearing the condom may be ready to go again after coming, after a bit of rest and further stimulation.

See section 4.12 for a suggestion about how to put a condom on.

Before putting the condom on. Make sure the penis is dry before you put the condom on, to reduce the risk of the condom slipping off. Avoid using, or carefully clean off, any kind of oil-based lubricant such as petroleum jelly or an oil-based massage cream or hand cream, because these substances can deteriorate the latex and cause a condom to break as well as slip.

Be sure that the penis and the hands of the person putting the condom on are clean of water-based lubricant as well, because this can cause the condom to slip if any gets between the penis and the inside of the condom.

If you have been enjoying oral sex just before putting on the condom, a quick wipe with a bed sheet or towel will remove any remaining saliva from the penis.

After the condom is on, a *water*-based lubricating jelly may be used on the outside of it, or on the person who will be penetrated. Common brands of "personal lubricants" are water-based and therefore safe to use with condoms. A condom that is dry on the outside can have difficulty entering, even if a woman has generated a fair amount of her own lubrication as she becomes aroused. For this reason it's good to have artificial lubricant available, at home or on a date, if you think you might be enjoying sex with a condom. Some condoms come pre-lubricated.

Checking during sex. It is a good idea to check periodically during genital or anal sex to be sure the condom has not slipped off. The man does not need to withdraw to do this; he can reach down with his fingers and feel for the ring around the opening of the condom. The person penetrated can also check in this way. The condom should be fully extended, so the ring is back near the base of the penis.

If the condom seems to be slipping a little, or in case of any doubt, either partner can hold the condom in place with thumb and forefinger on the ring while continuing normal in-and-out motions. If it's male-female genital sex, while the man is holding his thumb and forefinger on the condom ring in this way, with careful maneuvering he can also use his thumb to play with his partner's clit, which she will almost certainly appreciate along with the play of penis in vagina.

If the condom seems to be slipping a lot, it would be wise to withdraw for a moment, wipe the penis dry, and put on a fresh condom.

A broken condom is harder to detect without withdrawing completely. Since a man's feeling on his penis is usually noticeably different when wearing a condom than when he is not (he can feel the rubbing when not), a noticed difference in feeling is a clue for him that the condom may have broken or slipped off. If he thinks this might have happened, he should immediately withdraw momentarily to check. He should occasionally withdraw completely on general principles, just for a moment, even if he does not notice any difference in feeling, so he can visually check for possible condom rupture. This is especially a good idea just before he comes.

Withdrawing after ejaculation. After a man ejaculates and begins to lose his erection, the condom fits less snugly on him, so there is a greater chance that it will slip off as he withdraws. Of course he can withdraw immediately after ejaculation, before he begins to go soft, but this can be a jarring break of the blissful feeling of bondedness between the two partners that immediately follows orgasm. As an alternative, before or just as he starts to feel himself soften, he can reach down with thumb

4.04

and forefinger and hold the condom at its ring, keeping it in place. When he is ready to withdraw, he can continue holding the ring of the condom firmly to be sure that the condom comes out along with his penis. In any event, he should withdraw fairly soon after ejaculating.

When a condom breaks or slips off. If a condom breaks or slips off during sex with a secondary, it is important promptly to inform your primary partner(s) and any others with whom you are fluid-bonded. It would be courteous to inform as well any other secondary partners with whom you use condoms, since the risk to them is also increased at least slightly.

You can discuss with your fluid-bonded partner(s) the degree of risk that you feel has been incurred in the condom accident, and what measures you want to take. You may want to have yourself tested for STDs and ask the other person to be tested as well. Thorough testing would be once immediately and then again after the incubation period. See section 4.09 about getting tested and section 4.10 about the incubation period.

If you and your fluid-bonded partners decide that the incurred risk has been substantial, you may decide to use condoms with each other as a precaution until the incubation period has elapsed and you have tested clean thereafter (see section 4.13).

Sex during menstruation. Between fluid-bonded partners this is a matter of personal preference; the only reason not to share genital sex during menstruation is the mess that is created on your bodies and in the bed. For the bed, you can put down a large towel or the type of waterproof bed pad used in hospitals and nursing homes for incontinent patients. (See below in this section.)

When a man and woman use a condom and the woman is menstruating, there is a slightly greater risk of STD infection to the man, even with the condom, because the menstrual blood can spread above the top of the condom and onto other skin areas, where any slight break in his skin might allow entry of a microbe and infection.

I suggest that you discuss with your primary partner(s) whether or not sex with a female secondary will be allowed when the secondary is menstruating. You can then include this in your relationship agreement (see Chapter 5).

Waterproof pads. These pads have a waterproof backing on one side and comfortable absorbent padding on the other. They measure 85 × 72 centimeters, so one of them is normally big enough to catch any mess that two people can generate. If you roll around the bed a lot, or if there are more than two of you playing, you may want to put down more than one pad.

They are washable in a home laundry machine or coin machine.

These pads are also great not only for sex during menstruation but for women who "squirt" when they orgasm. The pads catch the "squirt" quite nicely.

Women, if you are prone to very heavy menstrual flow, and you occasionally leak onto the bed while you're sleeping, these waterproof pads will also catch your leak, preventing blood stains to sheet, mattress pad, or mattress.

To buy these pads, check with a pharmacy or look in the telephone yellow pages under "Hospital Equipment & Supplies". You will probably want several pads at least, so you will still have clean ones while some are in the laundry.

4.05. *Oral safe sex practices.*

Many people nonchalantly enjoy oral sex, giving and receiving, without being very concerned about possible disease transmission; and then they or their partner cautiously don a condom when they are ready for genital sex.

4.05

There is some indication that unprotected oral sex may be *somewhat* less risky than unprotected genital sex, especially for the "receiver" (the person whose genitals are licked and sucked), because saliva and gastric juices are able to destroy some microbes. However, the limitation of this rationale becomes obvious when you remember the rule you were taught as a child (and rightly so), and reminded of in every restroom in a restaurant or grocery store, always to wash your hands before eating or working with food. Germs can get transferred from a dirty hand to food to mouth and stomach, and you can easily get sick that way. So, germs can also get into your mouth from other body parts, and survive.

Not only that, but people commonly have skin breaks on the inside of their mouths of which they are unaware. People sometimes bite the inside of their cheeks in sleep or when eating, enough to break the skin. When you brush your teeth, does what you spit out into the sink sometimes have a pinkish tinge? Bleeding gums are common, especially when habits of brushing and flossing teeth are less than ideal. As with any other skin break, when blood can get out, nasty bugs can get in.

Even if there is no skin break inside the mouth, the skin in that area can be thin enough for some STD microbes to gain entrance.

See the descriptions of specific STDs in section 4.14 for discussion of how some STDs, normally infecting the genital area, can not only be transmitted by unprotected oral sex but can also produce unpleasant symptoms in the mouth and throat.

We might go on by mentioning peptic ulcers as another type of risky lesion—but of course you get the idea by now. Oral sex does involve some risk of infection. Just factor all this into your decision about whether the degree of risk in oral sex with someone new is acceptable.

Condoms for oral sex with a female receiver do exist, including those made of polyurethane for those allergic to latex. Other options for protection when giving oral sexual pleasure to a woman are to use a piece of plastic kitchen wrap, or cut the tip off a male condom with scissors and then cut it lengthwise, to create a flat sheet.

4.06. Anal safe sex practices.

Medical consensus is that unprotected anal sex (with penetration, or licking around the opening) is the riskiest form of sex, because the rectum has far more bacteria and viruses than the vagina, penis, or mouth. Thus, there is high risk of infection from the receiver to the giver (from the "bottom" to the "top"). The bottom is also at risk of infection, of course, from the top's ejaculate.

If you enjoy this form of sexual expression, with anyone other than a fluid-bonded partner who has tested clean and engages in no risky behavior with anyone else, be especially careful always to use a condom.

Always discard the condom and put on a fresh one before moving from anal penetration to vaginal.

4.07. Dildos, vibrators, and other sex toys.

Any such objects that are exposed to bodily fluids can become disease carriers. The best practice, therefore, is never to share these toys. If you do use sex toys with different partners who are not all fluid-bonded, wash them thoroughly between uses.

Another good practice with a dildo or other penis-shaped object that is shared is to cover it with a condom. A condom on a dildo or on a cucumber might even help it seem more realistic!

Is this too obvious to need mentioning? If a condom-covered toy is to be passed around, change the condom for each person!

4.08. Starting condom use after going condomless for a while.

Suppose you have had a somewhat casual sexual relationship for a while with someone (A), and you have not bothered using condoms with A. Now you are having second thoughts about how wise this is. Or maybe another relationship of yours (with B) is becoming stronger to the point where you and B are thinking about becoming primary and fluid-bonded, and as you and B are discussing what your safe sex practices with others will be, B says they are uncomfortable with your continuing to go condomless with A.

Is there any point in starting to use condoms with A now, or would that be a futile gesture, since you've already gone skin-to-skin with A for a while?

Yes, it is better to start condoms late than never. If A has an STD that you have not yet caught through sheer good luck, of course condoms will still offer you the same degree of protection against catching the disease in the future as if you'd been using condoms all along. Even if you *have* caught A's STD, using condoms with A from now on is still wise because A might pick up a different STD infection from a different partner of theirs.

You and B (as your primary) can consider continuing not to use condoms with A, if you and B wish, under the same criteria as you would use for a potential new secondary. See section 4.11 about fluid-bondedness.

4.09. Getting tested.

The importance of regular testing. As section 4.14 reflects, many people infected with any of several STDs never experience symptoms but are nevertheless contagious. Sometimes symptoms are rather mild so that an infected person might overlook them. For these reasons it is especially important for anyone who is sexually active, other than in a monamorous or polyfidelitous relationship in which all partners are known to be disease-free, to obtain regular across-the-board STD testing.

How often. For those who engage in light to moderate amounts of sex with different partners, being careful to use condoms and being choosy about partners, current medical consensus at this writing is to have an across-the-board STD testing about once a year. Check with your health care provider for possible updates. Your own chosen interval for routine STD testing can vary depending on your circumstances and what your health care provider recommends.

If there has been a condom accident with you or with a fluid-bonded partner of yours, or if there's been some other potential exposure, you may want to be tested promptly, regardless of how recently was your last testing. However, remember that negative testing results are not indicative until after the incubation period for each disease has expired (see sections 4.10 and 4.14).

If you and your primary partner(s) have gone for a long time with no new partners and no accidents, you may decide to defer testing somewhat beyond the recommended one-year interval. Of course, if in *any* doubt, get tested sooner rather than later.

Where. In North America, city and county health departments commonly provide STD testing services, generally without charge, with methods in place to protect your privacy and confidentiality. There are also nongovernmental clinics, such as Planned Parenthood. Phone your health department or similar agency in your area to see if they do testing, or to get a referral. If you have a primary care physician or a gynecologist, they should also be able to test you or give you a referral.

4.10. The incubation period.

The "incubation period" is the time between when a microbe first infects someone's body and when symptoms of disease typically first appear or when the disease can first be detected by medical tests. Each infectious disease, from the common cold to HIV, has its own incubation period, and the lengths of these periods vary widely from disease to disease, and sometimes from person to person. The incubation period for many STDs is included in the list of STDs in section 4.14.

The incubation period is a serious problem with all infectious diseases, STDs included, because a person can usually transmit a disease on to others during this time, when there are no symptoms and no other physical clues that the person is contagious, so the person genuinely believes they are disease-free, and even medical testing will not reveal the presence of the disease.

The incubation period is relevant to STD testing because a test will inaccurately give a negative result (no disease found) after infection but before the incubation period runs its course. This means that if you or someone close to you feel that you might have been exposed, you might want to be tested immediately on general principles, but you should also be tested again after the longest incubation period has lapsed. At this writing, the longest incubation period is for HIV, and is considered to be six months. (See the entry for "HIV" in section 4.14 for further discussion of the HIV incubation period.) Of course, testing sooner than six months—say, after a month or two or three—might bring to light another disease with a shorter incubation period.

If there has been a possible exposure, of course be extremely careful always to use protection during sex, or refrain, until you test clean after the incubation period. You and your (normally) fluid-bonded partner(s) might also consider using protection with each other during this time (see section 4.13).

4.11. *Criteria for fluid-bondedness.*

How safe is safe? It is personal preference how "clean" and "safe" a new sex partner must be before you agree to become fluid-bonded with them. If you already have one or more fluid-bonded partners (primary or secondary), then *all* those who are already fluid-bonded together should decide together about whether to add another person to the fluid-bonded group, since all will be sharing the risk more or less equally.

A reasonable minimum for allowing fluid-bondedness would be recent testing with negative results (that is, no diseases found), with no possible exposures during the incubation period (section 4.10) preceding the testing, and none since testing. If the potential new fluid-bonded partner is already fluid-bonded with one or more others, then of course the criterion for testing and lack of exposure applies to all who are fluid-bonded together with the potential new fluid-bonded partner.

You may also wish to consider the number of other sexual partners (even with condom use) that your proposed new fluid-bonded partner has. Since a condom does not totally eliminate risk of STD (accidents happen), you can think of the total degree of risk from a person as essentially the sum of the risks from each of their other partners. The more different partners that person has, the riskier that person is for you, with or without condoms.

You may also want to consider how careful the person in question is about sharing sex only with reasonably safe other partners. If someone is quick to share sex with someone new, with little or no inquiry as to their new partner's state of health, even though they always use condoms, you may consider this person too risky for yourself (and your fluid-bonded partners), even with condoms.

If there is any doubt or question in your mind, pull out a condom, or say, "Thanks, but no thanks."

4.12

Agreements with fluid-bonded secondaries. If you and your *primary* partner(s) decide to allow fluid-bondedness between any of you and a particular *secondary* partner, the secondary should agree not to go condomless with any new partner without prior agreement of *all* who are fluid-bonded together, and to let you know promptly not only of any infection to any of those fluid-bonded, but also if there is any accidental exposure with someone not fluid-bonded, as from a condom breaking or slipping off. Stress the importance of this agreement to the secondary. Obviously you should consider this option only if you trust the secondary's honesty 100%. You may want to consider the secondary's failure to abide by this to be automatic grounds to use condoms thereafter (if the relationship is continued).

4.12. *Making safe sex more fun.*

There is no avoiding the fact that using a condom detracts somewhat from the overall sexual experience. The feeling is not quite as good (especially for a man) as skin on skin. Stopping in the middle of passionate sex play to put on a condom can partially break the mood, at least for a moment.

There are some ways to alleviate this. You can have the condom out and within easy reach from the bed for when the time comes, maybe partially unwrapped in advance, so you don't need to rummage in a drawer or your pants pockets or purse or get up out of bed to find one. (Now where did I throw my pants, and which pocket did I stuff those condoms into?)

Many couples find that it adds to the sexual enjoyment, rather than detracting, when the man's partner puts the condom on for him. You and your partner may be able to invent games or rituals to add to the fun and lessen the distraction.

4.12

There are also faster and slower, more fun and less fun ways to get a condom on. The faster the better, I feel—unless you have discovered some way of making that process itself sexually stimulating. The standard method that I learned as a young man is to place the rolled-up condom, being careful that it's in the correct orientation, on the tip of the erect penis, then press down so as to unroll the condom onto the penis. Preparing to put on my own condom in that traditional manner, I am sometimes unsure that the condom is oriented correctly on the tip of my penis, especially in dim light; and sometimes I have a little trouble getting the condom started unrolling, coming up over the head of my penis.

One day a secondary lover showed me a fast and reliable way to get the condom on. It was more fun for both of us, too, since she got to slide her fingers along my hard penis as she did this.

Holding the unwrapped condom between thumb and forefinger in one hand (and being sure the orientation was right for unrolling), she held her two hands palms up, with the tips of her two index fingers pressed together, nail to nail. She then used her two thumbs to unroll the condom down over both index fingers together as if they were a penis, down to about the first joint. Getting the condom started unrolling over her fingers was much easier than unrolling it directly over my penis, since the two fingers together were a considerably smaller diameter than my penis.

With the condom partially unrolled in this way on her fingers, she then quickly pulled her index fingers apart, stretching the condom sideways and creating a gap the diameter of my penis, and then she brought her fingers, with the condom stretched between them, down the side of my penis, as far as it would go so as to avoid an air pocket. She then withdrew her fingers, and *voilà!* The condom was on me, about half unrolled. A quick stroke or two finished unrolling the condom, and we were ready to continue our fun. This whole process only took a couple of seconds.

A man can use this method on himself as quickly and easily as his partner can do it for him.

By the way, guys (and lovers who put the condoms on for your guys), have you ever paused to figure out which way condoms are oriented in their envelope? If you're at all like me, your mind is not thinking of that question when you rip open that envelope and pull the condom out of it! Then you have to waste a few seconds figuring out which way to position the condom so it will unroll.

At least with the brand that I usually use (is there an industry standard?), the condom will come out of its envelope with the correct side facing up for unrolling (assuming your hard cock—or your lover's—is pointing up) if the *back* side of the envelope is facing up as you pull the condom out of it.

Why the back side? There's a good question for the manufacturer; I have no idea.

Pleasure without penetration. If circumstances are such that penile penetration even with a condom would not be wise, or is not what you want to do for any other reason, there are still other ways of giving each other erotic and sensuous pleasure. Fingers are always handy for this—but be careful, if either of you is a health risk, that the giver has no skin breaks, even small ones, on their fingers. If this is a concern, you can wear a medical rubber glove if available, or unroll a condom over a finger or two fingers, holding it in place with your thumb. You can also get finger-sized condom-like rubber coverings, called "cots". Ask at your pharmacy for "finger cots".

Men who have beards usually learn fairly soon (or their lovers tell them) how nice a beard can feel when stroked like a feather across a groin, abdomen, or breasts.

And of course there are real feathers, dildos, vibrators, cucumbers, bananas…. Use your imagination, and experiment.

A massage, anything from one body part (head, neck, feet) up to a full-body massage, is another very good way to help each other feel physically very nice, short of actual sexual involvement. Although a massage is rather one-sided, you can take turns, and even the one giving the massage usually obtains considerable pleasure from the skin-to-skin contact as well as from knowing how good the other person is feeling under the stroking fingers. (The "receiver" should give plenty of feedback about what feels good or not so good as they are receiving the massage, including plenty of "ooohs" and "aaahs".)

Having two or three massage "givers" to one "receiver", then taking multiple turns so everyone gets to receive, is also a lot of fun for all involved. Some local polyamory groups hold "sensuous massage" sessions, where those assembled divide into groups of four, and in each foursome three people massage the fourth, and the massaging may include sexual stimulation of breasts and genitals, if the receiver wishes, but only by the massage givers' hands and fingers. The massage session is repeated three more times so that everyone has a chance to receive.

4.13. Using condoms among primaries or other fluid-bonded partners.

If you experience a possible STD exposure with a secondary (say, a condom breaks or slips off), it is a good idea to ask the other person immediately about their state of health, how recently they've been tested, etc., if you don't already know this. If the other person has not been tested recently, it is reasonable to ask them to be tested now, as a favor to you as well as for their own sake. Promptly let everyone with whom you are fluid-bonded know what happened, and what you learned about the degree of risk that was incurred.

Depending on the degree of risk, you and your fluid-bonded partner(s) might decide, for the sake of caution, to use condoms among yourselves until the incubation period has elapsed and you can all get new testing with negative results.

In addition to a possible or confirmed new STD infection in one fluid-bonded partner, an outbreak of a pre-existing but dormant infection, such as herpes, is another reason for normally fluid-bonded partners to use condoms for the interim.

4.14. *List of STDs.*

This section alphabetically lists all significant sexually transmitted diseases (STDs), describing symptoms, methods of transmission, and treatment. The incubation period is given for some of them. Note that, as a general rule, bacterial diseases are curable through antibiotics; most viral diseases are not curable, though their symptoms (if any) can sometimes be alleviated through medications.

AIDS

The acronym stands for "acquired immune deficiency syndrome". AIDS is caused by the virus called HIV and is thought of as a later stage of the HIV infection. See the separate entry for "HIV" in this list for further discussion.

Bacterial vaginosis

This is one of four separate diseases lumped under the group name "vaginitis". Bacterial vaginosis can be transmitted through unprotected genital sex, meaning that the bacterium can also infect men.

In women the symptoms can include a heavy menstrual discharge; a discharge not during menstruation that is thin, clear or whitish, and that smells fishy; and pain, itching, or burning. There may also be no symptoms. Symptoms in men are rare.

It is treatable by any of several medications; or treatment may not be needed. Consult your physician or clinic.

Chlamydia

Chlamydia is a bacterial disease transmitted sexually or from mother to baby during birth. When it is transmitted by childbirth, the baby can be infected in the eyes, ears, and lungs. Other than during childbirth, there must be direct contact between penis and vagina for transmission.

Men and women both usually show no symptoms. When symptoms do occur, they usually appear within 7 to 30 days. Symptoms can include a discharge from the penis, vagina, or rectum. Women may experience cramps or pain in the lower abdomen, and pain on urination. Men can have burning or itching around the opening of their penis, pain in the testicles, and pain on urination.

Because chlamydia is a bacterial disease, it can be cured with antibiotics.

If chlamydia is not promptly treated, it can lead to pelvic inflammatory disease (PID), tubal pregnancy, or infertility in women, and sterility or epididymitis in men. (See the separate entry for "Pelvic inflammatory disease" in this list.)

Clap, the

A colloquial term for gonorrhea; see the separate entry for "Gonorrhea" in this list.

Crabs

A colloquial term for pubic lice; see the separate entry for "Pubic lice" in this list.

Genital warts

These are small growths that typically appear on the outside of a man's penis or on and around a woman's vulva, inside her vagina, and around the cervical opening. Both men and women can also have genital warts in the throat or anus if they have shared unprotected oral or anal sex with an infected person. The warts can either be flat or appear as tiny bumps resembling cauliflowers. Sometimes they are too tiny to see with the naked eye. The only way to detect genital warts inside the vagina or anus and perhaps the throat is by a medical examination.

First symptoms typically appear after about 3 weeks, but in some cases after months or years.

Genital warts are caused by some varieties of the human papilloma virus (HPV). See the separate entry in this list for "Human papilloma virus".

Genital warts can be treated and removed by any of several methods, or they may spontaneously disappear. However, the HPV that causes them may remain in the body, and so, even if a particular outbreak of genital warts spontaneously disappears, it is important to get prompt medical treatment.

Gonorrhea

This disease is caused by a bacterial parasite and is transmitted via genital, oral, or anal sex, or from mother to baby during childbirth. It is curable through antibiotics either by injection or pills. All fluid-bonded partners must also receive the treatment.

Symptoms for men include tender or swollen testicles, or a greenish or yellow stain on their underwear or a drip from the penis. Women can have a gray or yellow vaginal discharge, heavier and painful menstruation, bleeding after sex or spontaneously (between periods), pain or cramps in the lower abdomen, fever, or nausea. Women and men both may notice pain or burning when they urinate, and more frequent urination, discharge from the rectum, or sore throat with difficulty swallowing (especially if transmission occurred by oral sex). Both genders can get a reddened or sore throat if they contract gonorrhea in the throat from oral sex; or blood, pus, and rectal pain when they defecate, due to gonorrhea in the rectum contracted by unprotected anal sex.

The incubation period for symptoms is usually 2 to 21 days. However, a majority of women and many men never show symptoms.

If gonorrhea is not promptly treated, it can lead to pelvic inflammatory disease in women. (See the separate entry for "Pelvic inflammatory disease" in this list.) If left untreated for a very long time in men or women, it can travel through the blood and settle in other parts of the body, causing infections in the brain, heart, joints, and skin.

Hepatitis

"Hepatitis" is a general name for inflammation of the liver. There are several different varieties of hepatitis, known as hepatitis A, B, C, and D. Colloquially the diseases are also known as "hep A", "hep B", etc. Each variety is caused by a different virus. People with any variety of hepatitis are more at risk for liver cancer, cirrhosis, and other liver diseases. They should also avoid overtaxing their liver by use of alcohol or other drugs or by taking certain prescription or nonprescription medications (including certain herbal medications).

The hepatitis A virus is present in an infected person's feces for about three weeks (from two weeks before to one week after onset of symptoms, when there are symptoms), and so anal sex, especially without condom use, is one means of transmission. Hepatitis A can also be transmitted through food that has been handled by an infected person who has not thoroughly washed their hands after using the bathroom, and from raw or undercooked shellfish gathered from contaminated waters.

Symptoms of hepatitis A appear within 2 to 6 weeks. Symptoms include jaundice (yellowish skin and eyes), brown or tea-colored urine, light-colored feces, diarrhea, fever, loss of appetite, stomach pain, nausea, and chronic fatigue. About half of adults and nearly all children who contract hepatitis A show no symptoms—but all who are infected can transmit the disease.

Because the hepatitis A virus is present in the feces of recently infected persons, it is especially important for those who engage

4.14

in anal sex to use a condom. Everyone should be especially careful to wash hands after using the toilet or changing diapers, and before touching food or eating.

A vaccine exists for hepatitis A. As with all vaccines, you must be vaccinated before you are exposed. However, if you may have been exposed but have not been vaccinated, another medication, promptly taken, can reduce your risk of contracting hepatitis A.

Hepatitis B can be transmitted sexually, because the virus is present in blood (including menstrual blood), semen, and other bodily fluids. It can also be transmitted by sharing such items as toothbrushes, razor blades, or nail clippers; from mother to baby during childbirth; or via dirty needles used for drugs, tattooing, or body piercing. Hepatitis B can also be transmitted by an accidental stick from a medical needle or other sharp medical instrument, a risk for health care professionals. Unlike hepatitis A, hepatitis B is *not* transmitted from handling or sharing food or drink.

The incubation period for hepatitis B is between 2 and 6 months.

Most children and about half of adults who contract hepatitis B never show symptoms. When symptoms do appear, they can include fatigue, loss of appetite, fever, stomach pain, nausea or vomiting, jaundice (yellowish skin and eyes), dark urine, and light-colored feces.

A percentage of those infected with hepatitis B (and especially babies who contract it at birth) will become life-long carriers of the hepatitis B virus, capable of transmitting it to others (including sex partners) even when they are showing no symptoms. Carriers have a higher risk of contracting other liver disease, such as liver cancer or cirrhosis. Carriers should be under regular medical care.

There is a vaccine for hepatitis B, a series of three injections, but (as with other vaccines) it is not effective after a person has been infected with the disease. When a pregnant woman tests positive for hepatitis B, doctors like to vaccinate the baby, starting with the first injection immediately after birth. This usually but not always protects the baby from contracting the disease.

People often never show symptoms with hepatitis B; or they may show symptoms fairly quickly (4 to 12 weeks) or only after a very long time, sometimes as long as 20 years.

Symptoms can include extreme fatigue, fever, stomach pain, loss of appetite, nausea, vomiting, jaundice (yellowish coloring of the skin and eyes), dark-colored urine, and very light-colored feces.

When jaundice and dark urine appear in a person with hepatitis B, there is probably liver damage, including scarring, liver cancer, and other damage. This liver damage can be fatal.

Hepatitis C is found in the bodily fluids and tissues of infected persons. It is transmitted primarily through exposure to blood and blood products. In addition to exposure due to certain medical procedures such as transfusion or hemodialysis, hepatitis C can also be transmitted through any form of sex, from mother to baby during childbirth, and by drug users sharing dirty needles.

The incubation period for hepatitis C is usually 6 to 8 weeks, but this can vary. Many infected persons show no symptoms. When symptoms do appear, they can include jaundice, fatigue, stomach pain, loss of appetite, nausea, and vomiting.

There are medications for treating hepatitis C, but these are effective only with a minority of infected persons. Those diagnosed with hepatitis C should be vaccinated for hepatitis A and B.

Because hepatitis D is not known to be transmitted sexually, it is not discussed here.

Herpes

(Pronounced "HER-peez". Adjective: *herpetic,* "her-PET-ik".) There are two strains of virus called "herpes simplex virus", or HSV. The two strains are called simply HSV-1 and HSV-2. These two strains are also known respectively as "oral herpes" and "genital herpes". People often say simply "herpes" when it is clear from context that the genital variety, HSV-2, is meant.

Both varieties of the herpes virus, especially HSV-1, are very prevalent. HSV-1 is found in about 80% of the United States population, and HSV-2 is in about 20% of the same population. Furthermore, a substantial percentage of those infected do not know that they carry the virus, since symptoms can be very mild or nonexistent.

Both kinds of herpes can be transmitted via genital, oral, or anal sex, and also by kissing or other contact with an infected area of the body, as described below.

Some people are infected with either variety of herpes but never experience symptoms. Others may experience painful sores or blisters on or near their mouth, genitals, or anus—wherever they were exposed to the virus. Symptoms may also include fever, a general achy feeling, and swollen lymph glands.

So-called "fever blisters" and "cold sores" around the mouth are herpes sores, usually but not always oral herpes. A person may experience itching or tingling before a sore develops. After the sore develops, it oozes for a while, then forms a scab, and later disappears.

Symptoms usually appear (if at all) within 2 to 12 days after infection.

The herpes virus concentrates in large numbers at the site of these sores, from the first indication of a developing sore until the sore has healed completely. One way that the virus can be transmitted to another person—or to another site on the same person—is by direct contact between the infected site and the mouth, genital area, eyes, or any skin break. The virus can also be transmitted indirectly if (for example) fingers touch an infected site and then touch any of the above-mentioned sites of possible entry.

Herpes is not curable, although the sores disappear after a while. There are, however, antiviral medications that can reduce the pain and discomfort from the sores. These medications can also decrease the frequency of outbreaks.

The virus then remains dormant in nerve cells close to where the sores were. A person may experience new outbreaks of sores at various intervals, or no recurrences at all. New outbreaks may be triggered by stress, or for no apparent reason. When recurrences do occur, sometimes they stop reappearing spontaneously later—although the herpes infection always remains dormant in the body. At this writing, medical science does not understand the reasons for these variations in how different people experience herpes.

After an outbreak of sores has disappeared, virus cells (residing in nearby nerve cells) can still travel back to nerve endings and out onto the skin surface, where the virus cells can remain without symptoms. Relatively few virus cells will be present on the skin surface when there are no visible sores, and so infection from this source is unlikely, although it does occasionally happen.

Herpes may or may not be transmitted from a pregnant woman to her fetus. Herpes can be transmitted to a baby during birth, but only if there is an active outbreak on the mother's skin at the time. For this reason, if a woman has an active herpes outbreak when she goes into labor, her attending physician may recommend a cesarean. Thus, if you are pregnant and if you have ever had "cold sores" or any other kind of herpes outbreak, it is important to let your physician know.

The best protection against spreading herpes (second to abstention) is to avoid touching any herpes sore, or spot where a sore appears to be developing, on yourself or on a sexual partner. If the outbreaks are in the genital area of either one of you, use condoms, even with those with whom you are normally fluid-bonded.

HIV

The acronym stands for "human immunodeficiency virus". HIV gradually reduces and ultimately destroys a person's natural immune system (or "autoimmune system"), the body's natural ability to fight off infectious diseases.

4.14

First symptoms may appear within a few weeks. Symptoms can include fatigue, weight loss, diarrhea, and recurrent infections; or there may be no symptoms.

A later stage of the HIV infection, after the immune system has been seriously damaged, is called "AIDS" ("acquired immune deficiency syndrome"). AIDS is also listed separately above, since it is sometimes thought of as a disease in its own right, but this discussion here of HIV includes a more complete discussion of AIDS.

HIV stays in bodily fluids, such as vaginal fluids, semen, and blood, and so it can be transmitted during oral, genital, or anal sex. It can also be transmitted via dirty needles used medically or used for drugs, body piercing, or tattooing. The virus is found also in mother's breast milk, and so it can be transmitted to a baby via breastfeeding as well as during pregnancy or childbirth. Since 1985, blood donated for transfusion is always carefully tested for HIV (as well as other possible diseases), and so blood received in a transfusion is extremely safe.

A bright spot is that HIV will not inhabit *all* bodily fluids. In particular, HIV cannot be transmitted through saliva, sweat, tears, or urine. Solid objects, such as toilet seats, telephones, eating utensils, or towels, also cannot transmit HIV.

There is no cure for HIV, including the AIDS phase. The HIV/AIDS combination is considered generally fatal, although people usually die not from AIDS itself but from so-called "opportunistic diseases". As the full names of both acronyms suggest, HIV and AIDS steadily break down the human body's normally very effective immune system, so that other infectious diseases (such as pneumonia or tuberculosis), normally treatable and curable, can more and more easily take the opportunity to infect that person; and, after infection, the normal treatments for those other diseases are not effective. Because the body is weaker in general than normal, these opportunistic diseases then can manifest with symptoms much more powerful and destructive than usual, leading ultimately to death.

A person who is HIV-positive (or HIV+), meaning that the virus has been found in their body, can sometimes go for years after infection with no feeling of being sick and no apparent symptoms. HIV/AIDS is usually detectable three months after infection, but sometimes the delay before detectability may be as long as six months, and so six months is considered the standard incubation period for HIV. This is by far the longest incubation period of any STD. Therefore, if you think there is even a slight chance that you might have been exposed to HIV, you should be tested now, and again after three months. If the three-month test shows negative, get yourself tested one more time after three additional months.

Human papilloma virus (HPV)

HPV is spread during unprotected sex, and there is no cure. There are several varieties of HPV. One variety causes genital warts (see "Genital warts" listed separately above). Some other varieties never show symptoms but are linked to higher risk of cervical cancer. All varieties, including those causing genital warts, can sometimes be present without symptoms, so the disease can be transmitted by people who do not know that they are infected. The higher-risk varieties of HPV can often be detected by Pap tests, which is one important reason for women to have those tests at the recommended intervals.

Molluscum contagiosum

This is a viral infection. Symptoms of skin-colored bumps and itchiness may appear after one week to six months.

The symptoms may disappear spontaneously. A treatment can destroy the viral core.

Nongonococcal urethritis (NGU)

As the name implies, this is an inflammation of the urethra (the tube by which urine leaves the body). It is transmitted by genital sex. Symptoms appear within 7 to 21 days. Men and women both may experience pain or discomfort on urination. Men may notice a discharge from the penis (sometimes this is noticed only in the morning). NGU can lead to infection in other reproductive organs.

4.14

NGU can by cured by proper medical treatment. Notify recent sex partners that they should see a doctor. Refrain from sex until you and your partners are cured.

Pelvic inflammatory disease (PID)

PID is not strictly speaking an STD, but we will list it here because the vast majority of cases are caused by STDs. Various STDs can lead to PID, but the most common are gonorrhea and chlamydia.

PID is an infection of a woman's reproductive organs. It can lead in turn to serious problems in those reproductive organs, including difficulty in getting pregnant, ectopic pregnancy, or infertility. Aside from the symptoms of the STD that led to PID, symptoms of PID itself can be one or any number of the following, or there can be no symptoms: painful or heavy menstruation; vaginal bleeding when not menstruating; other abnormal vaginal discharge; pain or cramps in the lower abdomen; lower back ache; pain during urination and during sex; nausea or vomiting; fever.

The majority of cases of PID occur in young women, including teenagers, who are sexually active and not cautious about sexual hygiene, because the adolescent female reproductive organs are not yet fully mature and have less resistance to infection.

The incubation period for PID is between several days and several months from the date of contracting the STD that leads to PID, the specific period depending on the STD and on the individual's resistance.

Although men cannot contract PID, they can of course contract the STDs that lead to PID in their female partners. Not only that, but men are somewhat more likely than women to experience symptoms of the STDs that lead to PID in women. This is one more reason why any hetero or bi man who discovers or suspects that he might have an STD should have that checked out immediately; and he should inform his female partner(s) of his condition.

PID can be cured with antibiotics, but any woman who suspects that she might have PID should see her physician promptly. It may not be possible to reverse damage already done to a woman's reproductive system if the disease has progressed that far. Once a woman has had a case of PID, she is more likely to contract it again.

If a woman is diagnosed with PID, all her fluid-bonded partners need to be treated with her, to prevent the disease from being passed back and forth. It is best in this case for the fluid-bonded partners to refrain from sex until the disease is cleared up, or (second best) scrupulously use condoms during the interim.

Some medical researchers suspect that there is higher risk of PID when a woman has an intrauterine device (IUD) installed. Therefore, if you are diagnosed with an STD, be sure to let your doctor know if you have an IUD installed.

PID

The acronym stands for "pelvic inflammatory disease". See the separate entry for "Pelvic inflammatory disease" in this list.

Pubic lice

These are a parasitic species of insect that infect a person's pubic area, and so these lice can be transferred from one person to another during genital sex (and condoms are *not* a protection against them, since they can jump from one pubic area to another when in proximity). Once a person is infected, the lice can also infest clothing, upholstered furniture (including in a car), and carpeting, and this can also lead to transmission even without sex.

Symptoms appear after 7 to 30 days, and include intense itching and tiny blood spots on underwear after the underwear is worn. You may also notice lice and their eggs in your pubic hair.

Your doctor can prescribe a treatment to rid you of the lice.

Wash or dry-clean any clothing worn before starting the treatment, and also wash your bed linens. Thoroughly vacuum your sofa and any upholstered chairs, your mattress, your carpeting, and your car seats and carpeting.

Inform any recent sex partners that they should see a doctor.

Scabies

The scabies mite is another parasite, like pubic lice. Condoms do *not* provide protection. The incubation period and symptoms are somewhat different from those of pubic lice, however. Symptoms of scabies usually appear in 2 to 6 weeks (or within one to four days if re-exposed). Symptoms include intense itching, especially at night, and raised lines on the skin in areas where the mites burrow—genitals, breasts, hands, buttocks, or abdomen.

Your doctor can prescribe a treatment to rid you of the scabies mite.

Wash or dry clean any clothing worn before starting the treatment, and also wash your bed linens. Thoroughly vacuum your sofa and any upholstered chairs, your mattress, your carpeting, and your car seats and carpeting.

Inform any recent sex partners that they should see a doctor.

Syphilis

(Adjective: *syphilitic*.) Syphilis is a disease caused by a bacterium and is spread via genital, oral, or anal sex. It can also be transmitted from mother to baby during childbirth. Babies infected in this way can be stillborn or, if born alive, they can have liver failure; damage to brain, eyes, bones, teeth, and skin; pneumonia; and bleeding. Babies born alive with syphilis often die soon after birth.

Some people never notice symptoms. It can be detected by medical test after the incubation period of one to three weeks (occasionally longer). It can also be detected after symptoms have disappeared (as described below). It is curable with antibiotics, either an injection or longer treatment.

Syphilis occurs in three distinct phases. When symptoms do appear, the first phase can include one or a number of sores called "chancres" (pronounced "SHANK-ers"). The size of a chancre can vary from around 3 millimeters to 40 millimeters in diameter. Chancres may be accompanied by sore and swollen lymph nodes in the vicinity, but chancres themselves are usually painless.

Chancres will disappear after another one to eight weeks. Because an infected person may experience only one chancre (typically near the part of the body where infection occurred—genitals, mouth, or rectum), and the chancre may be small and because it disappears in time, the infected person may not notice it or may not realize that it is a serious problem. The infection remains (if untreated), and other symptoms can appear later in the second phase, including flu-like symptoms, fever, headaches and other aches, sore throat, loss of appetite, weight loss, swollen glands, or skin rash in various areas or all over.

These second-stage symptoms also disappear in time, even if the disease is not treated. After further time, more serious problems start to appear, including swollen glands, hair loss, headache, and sore throat. The late stages of the disease can also bring permanent damage to the brain, heart, other body organs, bones, and skin.

As mentioned, syphilis is curable. If a person is not cured of it, the disease can lead to crippling, blindness, or insanity, and even death, even long after the person was infected.

Trichomoniasis

(Pronounced "trick-o-mo-NĪ-a-sis".) Colloquially it is also called "trich", pronounced like "trick". This is one of four separate diseases lumped under the group name "vaginitis"; however, it can also infect and affect men. It is usually transmitted via unprotected genital sex, but it can also be transmitted by sharing damp towels, underwear, or bathing suits.

Trichomoniasis is caused by a parasite. Symptoms usually appear between 5 and 28 days after infection. Symptoms in women can include vaginal burning or itching, or both; and a yellowish, greenish, or gray vaginal discharge that smells fishy. Men may experience severe irritation of the penis, including a burning sensation after urinating or ejaculating; and sometimes a mild discharge. Women and men both may also experience no symptoms. Trichomoniasis may lead to urinary tract infections.

Trichomoniasis in a pregnant woman can cause premature labor and low-birth-weight babies.

It is treated with antibiotics.

Vaginitis

This is a general term that covers four unrelated vaginal conditions. These are bacterial vaginosis, atrophic vaginitis, trichomoniasis, and yeast infections. Atrophic vaginitis is not transmitted sexually, and yeast infections usually are not. Since this chapter is about STDs, we will not discuss those two diseases here, other than to note that there are medications for treating them.

Since bacterial vaginosis and trichomoniasis can be transmitted sexually, they each have entries in this list.

Vaginosis

See "bacterial vaginosis" in this list.

Yeast infections

Not usually transmitted sexually. See under "vaginitis".

~ 5 ~
The Relationship Agreement

Contents:
5.01. Who needs an explicit relationship agreement?
5.02. When to develop the agreement.
5.03. Written or oral?
5.04. What the relationship agreement should cover.
5.05. Modifying the relationship agreement.
5.06. Sample agreement for a dyad.

♥ ♥ ♥

5.01. Who needs an explicit relationship agreement?

Society's norms. Every society, ours no exception, has assumed norms of behavior that are so deep-rooted that they are unwritten and largely unconscious. Our laws and religious teachings reflect them; they do not create them.

Some of these norms make good sense—some variation of the Golden Rule, for example—and some of them are . . . well, quaint. If anthropologists discovered a hitherto unknown tribe on an isolated island who followed some of our customs, we would exchange superior smiles with each other at the wonder that some people could be so primitive as to live that way. If a delegation from that tribe were brought to North America or Europe to learn how we live, they would probably give each other the same superior smiles over some of what *we* do.

5.01

In our own society, as we know (when we think about it consciously), the norms that pertain to interpersonal relationships say that when boys and girls grow up they are expected to find one person of the other gender to marry and raise children with. After they find their one mate, they are supposed to lose all their biological sexual interest in anyone else; or if somehow they find themselves having the forbidden feelings, then they must suppress them, and certainly never act on them.

Following or diverging from the norms. A married man and woman in mainstream society—or a gay or lesbian couple who follow the same pattern except for gender—may feel that they do not need an explicit relationship agreement that just restates the norms; they already know how everyone is supposed to behave. Even for them, though, a relationship agreement can be quite useful, as many relationship professionals are now coming to recognize and recommend. The contents of their mainstream relationship agreements, of course, will not contain provisions pertaining to conduct of secondary relationships. But as soon as two or more people decide to live their lives together in some sexually nonstandard way, it needs to be a conscious, explicit decision, including provisions about sexual behavior; and an explicit statement of the particulars of their decision (sexual or otherwise) becomes far more important and useful.

Some might say, if a couple decides explicitly to live polyamorously, isn't that enough? Many (maybe even most) poly couples, triads, etc., think so, and do not bother to develop a "relationship agreement" as such, whether written out or not. My own experience is, however, that an explicit relationship agreement can head off many misunderstandings and disagreements, and greatly alleviate those that do arise.

If polyamory consisted simply of a single alternative norm—maybe along the lines that "multiple sexual relationships are okay as long as everyone concerned is open, honest, and in agreement"—then, again, a relationship agreement would be less useful, since the alternative norm would be easy enough to keep in mind. But, as we all know, polyamory is infinitely varied, because all details are open to separate choice.

For these reasons I strongly recommend that *every* primary couple or group practicing any form of polyamory should have an *explicit* relationship agreement, reflecting their preferences on the points covered.

Section 5.03 discusses whether the agreement should be written or oral.

For secondary relationships, the benefits of a relationship agreement are less obvious, and most secondary relationships can probably do well without one—although secondary partners certainly should come to some understandings, such as safe sex practice with each other and/or others; under what circumstances the wishes of the secondary partners should yield to the primary relationships that any of them are in; how much and what sort of information is to be shared between them and with others; etc. Having a relationship agreement is always an option in secondary relationships, especially those that are deeper and more involved.

An explicit relationship agreement certainly is no guarantee against disagreements or misunderstandings. For one thing, there are always gray areas, and different people can interpret a word or phrase in an agreement differently, as we all know. For another, we cannot anticipate everything that might come up in life. (Wouldn't life be dull if we *could* anticipate everything?)

So, even with a relationship agreement, you can expect to have occasional discussion with your primary partner(s) on how to proceed about something, and you are likely to find things you want to add or modify based on your ongoing experience.

5.02. When to develop the agreement.

Let's suppose that you are in a new and rising polyamorous relationship (dyad, triad, or more), and you have high hopes that it will develop all the way to become primary. Or, suppose you have been in a sexually exclusive couple relationship for some time, and the two of you have recently agreed to try polyamory. Or, your couple relationship has been polyamorous for some time, and the two of you have managed fine so far without an explicit relationship agreement. When should you consider developing such an agreement?

The general suggestion here is, the earlier the better when you think of yourselves as primary with each other and your relationship is polyamorous.

New primary couples or groups. If you are experienced with polyamory but you and your partner(s) are just starting to think of yourselves as primary, developing your relationship agreement now will have at least two benefits. It will help you focus on a number of questions which you need to decide between you as you embark on a polyamorous life together, some of which you might not happen to think of otherwise. It will also help prevent you from falling inadvertently into any habits that might lead to misunderstandings and disagreements later.

It could possibly even bring to light some areas of basic incompatibility that may cause you both to rethink the wisdom of becoming primary. It would be better to discover these things now than after your lives have become more enmeshed with each other.

Established couple new to polyamory. If you are an established couple but both of you are new to polyamory (or to having an open relationship of any sort), it is especially important for you to become aware of and consider the various questions on which you will need to reach agreement in order to give yourselves the best odds of smooth sailing and greatest satisfaction.

In your situation as an established couple, the two of you already have established habits of relating with each other. Some of these habits are universal and will continue to be important (mutual trust, flexibility, empathy, sense of humor, and others), but some habits will probably need to be changed (automatically panicking if your partner shows interest in someone else, feeling reluctance about expressing to your partner your own warm feelings for someone else). You will both need to stay alert to the changed, unfamiliar ways of relating, until they in turn become second-nature to you both.

You have lived in a primary polyamorous relationship for some time without an explicit relationship agreement. It could be that the two of you are naturally very closely attuned to each other, so that you just naturally tend to come to the same ideas and feelings without needing much explicit discussion (what is sometimes called a "low-maintenance relationship"). This is wonderful if true—but beware of the possibility that one of you might be consciously or subconsciously setting aside your own preferences and desires for any of a number of psychological reasons, thereby giving a false impression of unanimity. If this is the case, then the one of you who is putting yourself down and submitting to the other's wishes needs to work on improving your self-image and assertiveness, and then later come back to formulating your relationship agreement.

Even if the two of you are genuinely in good resonance with each other, and you have lived together for some time as polyamorous primaries without an explicit relationship agreement, it is still a good idea to make your agreement explicit now. You may find that there are some points on which you *thought* the two of you agreed, but upon discussion you learn that you are not quite that unanimous after all. You may have good agreement on broad principles (say, using condoms with anyone else) but you may discover disagreements on some of the finer points (say, whether or how to exercise judgment about when it is safe to make an exception and forego the condoms).

5.03. Written or oral?

You both may feel that for something so basic to your primary relationship as your relationship agreement, you will both remember the details of your agreement without needing to commit it to paper. Putting the relationship agreement in writing may seem contentious or legalistic.

Unfortunately, people have a tendency, even with the best of good will, to perceive and remember things selectively and with a slant more in line with their own individual preferences and views of reality. In the case of relationship agreements, this phenomenon tends to come to light a while later when there is an exchange something like this: "Say, honey, why did you do X, when we agreed that we wouldn't do that?" "Oh, but I thought we agreed that X was okay!" Or, "Well, the way *I* understand X, what I was doing was not X, so I felt I was carefully abiding by our agreement!"

Putting your agreement in writing will not guarantee freedom from misunderstandings or different interpretations of a word or phrase, but it does guarantee freedom from forgetfulness, and the disputes that result. This factor alone makes the effort of putting the agreement down on paper worthwhile. ("Why are you saying that I went against our agreement? I don't think we agreed to anything of the sort." "Sorry, honey, but right here it is, third paragraph on page 2!" "Gosh, you're right. Okay, I apologize for my forgetfulness. I won't do that again, I promise.")

The agreement itself of course will speak in generalities, but it is very helpful for avoiding future differences of interpretation, as you are discussing and formulating each provision of your agreement, to think up illustrative hypothetical examples as a sort of "practice" application of each provision. If you find differences between you when you do this, you will want to either find different wording for the ambiguous phrase or add text to clarify what you do agree to, more specifically. ("Okay, honey, this sentence in our draft says, 'Neither of us will share sex with anyone else in our own bed.' Let's suppose that Jane and I go off for a camping weekend, and we take the tent and camping equipment that you and I have. Does the phrase 'our own bed' apply also to our air mattress and double sleeping bag?" "Good question—I didn't think of that. Hmmm. Thinking about that possibility, I don't think it would bother me. It's just our bed at home that I'm sentimental about." "So then, how about if we change 'our own bed' in the agreement to read 'our own bed *at home*'? Or add a sentence, 'This does not apply to camping equipment.'" "Sure, either of those would fix it.")

5.04. *What the relationship agreement should cover.*

The agreement *can* cover anything between you (pertaining to polyamory or not) when you feel it is important to establish agreement in advance. As a practical matter, for polyamorous couples or larger primary groups, certain elements stand out either as universal, or should at least be considered for inclusion. This section lists many such questions, as suggestions for you to consider, first as to whether to include the topic, and second as to what your agreement on that topic will be.

The questions are in italics. In plain text I offer my own comments. How you decide them and phrase your answers in your relationship agreement is, of course, entirely up to you, since it's a matter of your preferences. There is no order of importance to the following list.

5.04

a. *May either of us have one or more outside personal relationships that could include sex?* If "yes", this basically establishes that the primary relationship is polyamorous—or at least is sexually open in some way. For triads and up, if the answer is "no", this means that the group is adopting polyfidelity—which is considered to be a variety of polyamory. For polyfidelitous groups, many of the following questions, pertaining to secondary relationships, will drop out of consideration.

b. *For a triad or larger, how do we decide sleeping arrangements or sex partners for a given night?* In some triads, for example involving three heterosexuals sharing a single king-size bed, this is not a question; the two partners of the same gender will typically be on the outside. When I lived in a quad (all four of us hetero), one of the four of us would invite a bed partner for the night at some point before bedtime. We usually alternated, but not always.

c. *Do we set a maximum number of secondaries that we each may have at one time?* The larger the number of secondaries, the more difficult it will be to juggle scheduling and prevent the secondary relationships from interfering in the primary relationship. The intensity of secondary relationships will have the same effect. Having more secondaries also increases STD risk somewhat, even with condom use. However, you may not need to fix a numerical limit in your relationship agreement; as each primary adds new secondary relationships, or as any secondary relationship comes to consume more time and energy, you are likely to notice as it becomes awkward to add another one.

d. *How much of a say, if any, does one of us have in approving a secondary partner for the other of us?* This can vary from complete

5.04

"veto power" to complete freedom. Intermediate positions could include offering one's candid opinion of a secondary or would-be secondary, with the other partner promising to consider the offered opinion carefully but still retaining the right to decide. Factors that can lead one to prefer a greater say on this question are a tendency to jealousy, less than total trust in a primary partner's judgment in making wise decisions, and having a general desire for control over other people as part of one's personality—or simply being new to polyamory and wanting to take things slowly, which of course is sensible. "Veto power" or something approaching it could be useful at least as an initial position when a couple is first becoming accustomed to polyamory; they might consider relaxing their agreement on this question later, after they've gained some experience.

e. *How much information do we give each other about each secondary relationship or partner, and about our own feelings about that relationship?* The common-sense rule widely followed in polyamory is that the more information shared, the better. An extreme can include giving each other copies of all email and online chats with the secondary, and giving a general summary of phone calls or other voice conversations. The opposite extreme is "don't ask, don't tell", by which it is agreed that each primary may have secondary relationships, as long as they don't interfere with life in the primary relationship, but neither partner will offer any information at all even about whether they have any secondary relationships currently, nor ask their primary for any such information. Some might think of the "don't ask, don't tell" option as a first step toward opening one's relationship, but be careful that it is not an attempt by either of you to avoid confronting deep-seated discomfort or insecurity in oneself about the basic polyamorous arrangement. If the latter is the case, it would probably be better to deal with those insecurities first, before attempting polyamory or any other form of open relationship. If you don't, the insecurities will very likely pop out later in unpleasant ways.

f. *May one of us go on dates with a secondary without the other of us present?* This is probably the most common way to conduct secondary relationships. If at least one member of a poly couple is bisexual, the two of them may simply prefer dating someone together, at least sometimes. On the other hand, if one primary partner is uncomfortable seeing the other primary head off with a secondary, this may be an indicator of jealousy or general lack of comfort with the basic polyamorous arrangement.

g. *May either of us stay away overnight with a secondary? Longer than one night?* This is largely a matter of personal comfort, but other factors could be whether the one(s) left at home must handle childcare or other home duties that would be doubled up when one is absent. I recall a conversation among a group in which my partner and I were the only polyamorous people present, and the others were all swingers. One woman asked the group how long people felt it was appropriate for someone to stay away with a different partner. She was thinking in terms of 45 minutes or an hour—long enough for a couple of orgasms in a back room at a party. She was astonished to hear my partner say she felt that a day or so was reasonable, unless the two primaries arranged for a longer absence with a secondary. But as with everything else, what matters here is what is comfortable for *each of you*.

h. *May we invite a secondary to our own home? If so, do we need to give advance notification by phone to anyone already at home that a guest will be arriving? May we share sex with a secondary in our own bed? Elsewhere in our home?* Some primary couples consider their own bed to be "special" to them, simply as a sentimental thing, or because of odors. If this is the case, preferring not to share sex with anyone else in that bed does not indicate jealousy or insecurity. Allowing sex with a secondary, or even sexual play such as fondling, in a commonly shared part of the home such as the living room, can raise questions when other family members are present or may return home. Does everyone give the lovers privacy, preventing others from using the living room or even walking through? One solution is to agree that if any primary partner engages in any sexual activity (with another primary or with anyone else) in a normally common area such as the living room or hot tub, then those so engaged tacitly agree that others may come and go, and there can be no expectation of privacy.

i. *Will we always use a condom with anyone other than each other?* Requiring a condom 100% of the time (when at least one partner is male) is obviously safest, but the price is losing the flexibility of allowing fluid-bondedness in a particular case that seems to pose acceptably low risk.

j. *If we allow the possibility of fluid-bondedness with a secondary, then must we agree between us, in advance, that a particular person is safe enough for condomless sex, or can each of us use our own best judgment with a new secondary partner as to whether to forego a condom?* This is essentially a matter of preference for the primary couple or group, and could depend on how well each primary partner trusts the other(s) to exercise good judgment, or just on how much they want decisions to be shared between them. The primary group might set up a list of criteria (say, recently testing negative and no recent risky behavior), which, if met, would allow one primary partner to proceed condomless without consulting the other(s) first.

k. *Regardless of our agreement regarding condoms, will we allow oral-genital sex with others?* Medical consensus is that there is rather less risk of STD transmission from the giver to the receiver of oral sex (regardless of the gender of the receiver), and so you may wish to consider allowing any party to this agreement to *receive* oral pleasure without protection as a default, unless there is a reason to the contrary, such as skin breaks, questionable personal history, etc. *Giving* oral pleasure without protection is somewhat riskier, since the giver will inevitably take in some of the receiver's bodily fluids, whether the receiver is male or female. Obviously the greatest exchange of fluids is when a male receiver ejaculates into the mouth of a giver. See section 4.05.

l. *Will we allow digital stimulation of another person?* This could be risky to the giver if the giver has skin breaks on the hand used for stimulation, unless a glove or condom is worn. There can also be risk to the receiver if the giver has a skin break on the active hand that results in bleeding.

m. *How often will we undergo STD testing?* Current medical consensus is that anyone sexually active with multiple partners should undergo STD testing at least once a year. If anything occurs to raise any question, such as a broken or slipped condom, or if you learn that someone that you (or anyone fluid-bonded) have recently shared sex with has been tested positive for some STD, then prompt new testing is a good idea, and again after the incubation period. See Chapter 4.

n. *Will we let our children know, to a degree commensurate with their level of maturity, that their parents are polyamorous?* This question is relevant only to polyamorous singles and couples. A triad or larger primary group is in effect declaring their polyamorous lifestyle to the children in their household and to the world continuously. Communicating with children is discussed in section 8.08.

o. *How do we deal with phone calls from secondaries to the home, or personal visits from secondaries to the home or with us elsewhere, when the children are also present?* If the decision to the previous question was to be open with the children, then this question is almost moot. Mom's on the phone with her special friend Bob. Dad will be going out this evening with his special friend Mary. A term like "special friend" is useful for children too young to understand romance and sex. From about puberty on through adolescence, it should be possible to explain and use common poly terminology, such as "secondary lover" or just "lover". If the primary group decides to hide their polyamory from the children, then they will need to devise circumlocutions (hopefully not lies) to tell the children. Again, see section 8.08.

p. *May any primary keep information confidential or secret from the other primary or primaries?* This could lead to problems; I feel it is important that all significant information be shared with all primaries. The only exception is temporary, to allow surprise birthday and holiday gifts and the like. However, all primaries may agree together to hold information confidential from others outside the primary group, if there is no ethical problem involved. This will protect the privacy of secondary partners, allow others to stay in the closet, etc.

q. *If our finances are partially shared and partially separate, how will dates with secondaries be paid for? Birthday and holiday gifts, etc., for secondaries?* This is really a matter of personal preference, but you should discuss it among you and agree on this in advance, to avoid misunderstandings and disputes. It might seem reasonable that dates with secondaries, when not all primaries are included, should be paid by the personal funds of those partners who are included. Similarly, how gifts are paid for might depend on whether they are to be given by all or fewer than all of the primary partners.

5.05. Modifying the relationship agreement.

Your couple or primary group will probably want to modify your relationship agreement as you gain experience living together with polyamory. If you are a couple just experimenting with opening your relationship, or if you are a new couple, triad, etc., not yet familiar with how each of you will react to various situations, you will probably want to err on the side of caution at first (for example, wanting to introduce any potential secondary partner to the other of you and then consulting between you before becoming sexually engaged). As you gain experience, you may find that you are comfortable relaxing some initial restrictions. You may also find that you need to clarify some ambiguity or difference of interpretation of a provision.

If you yourself have any questions or discomforts with how your relationship agreement is worded or how it is being observed by all of you, do not hesitate to ask for a "family discussion" (held lovingly and respectfully, of course) among both/all primaries to clarify the matter. All primaries should share their feelings fully.

See Chapter 6 about communication techniques and other relationship skills, and Chapter 7 regarding resolution of issues.

This discussion may result in agreement about how to interpret some provision, or you may decide, after discussion, that you need to add clarifying language or change some wording.

5.06. *Sample agreement for a dyad.*

What follows is the real relationship agreement that is in effect at this writing between myself and my primary partner, Deborah. This is certainly not the only possible format—it's your relationship and your relationship agreement!

Look at this sample and see if at least some parts of it seem to reflect the situation for you and your primary partner. If so, you could take this agreement, or parts of it, as a starting point, and then change, add, or delete language as you see fit.

♥ ♥ ♥

Relationship Agreement— Deborah & Pete

Emotional interactions

General. We recognize that any loving relationship requires continual positive nourishment to survive, thrive, and grow. With that in mind, we promise always to behave, whether we are together or apart, so as to reassure each other of our mutual love and emotional commitment. We agree always to share information and our feelings about each other, about other people, or about other aspects of our lives with complete openness and honesty. We will offer information to each other not only truthfully but completely, avoiding deliberate half-statements or "lies by omission" that might lead the other of us to incorrect inferences due to missing or incomplete information. We will continually reassure each other of our love and respect for the other. We will answer any questions from the other of us truthfully and completely (also with love and respect), and we will not hesitate to ask the other of us questions (also with love and respect).

Walking the path together. We recognize that a loving partnership represents a mutual agreement to help each other in our ongoing personal and spiritual growth. We recognize that a deficiency in either of us is not something to be criticized as a "fault" but is a weak area needing further development. Toward that end, we agree to help each other with love and respect to recognize those weak areas and to grow in them. We agree to be as totally open psychologically to each other as possible, and to lovingly hold up a mirror to each other so we may each better see into the subconscious and more hidden reaches of our own psyches, with the goal of continuing to learn and grow as long as we are together in this plane.

Primary status. We agree that our relationship with each other is primary. This means that we agree that we are open to additional friendships or loving relationships, with either gender, and including sexual expression if desired, but only as long as the additional relationship does not detract or threaten to detract from our own relationship. We agree that our own relationship will take priority over any other emotional, romantic, or sexual relationships that either of us may develop. In arranging times and activities with other friends or lovers, we will consult with each other so as to blend the outside activities with our own shared life as smoothly as possible. We will try to resolve any scheduling conflicts to everyone's satisfaction, but if it is impossible to accommodate everyone, then scheduling for each other, and nurturing our own relationship, will take priority over scheduling for one of us with another person.

Expression of anger. We promise not to let annoyances or anger toward the other of us fester or lie hidden, but always to express our feelings to each other fully and promptly. However, even in moments of anger or other negative feelings, we promise always to treat each other with the respect and courtesy that we each deserve, never putting the other down verbally or otherwise. In speaking with or writing to any third party, neither of us will ever use disrespectful or demeaning language about the other of us. We will never touch each other in any way other than loving.

Resolution of differences. We will always work promptly to resolve any disagreements that may arise. If either of us feels that it would be better to postpone discussion of a disagreement (for example, because of an angry mood or because of current circumstances), either of us may request deferment of the discussion and propose a specific time as soon as practicable to pick up the discussion again. We will not leave a disagreement unresolved unless either we have agreed to a time to resume the discussion or we have "agreed to disagree", i.e., we have agreed to live with the difference indefinitely with no further attempt to come to agreement.

Mutual support. We agree to help, support, and comfort each other in any personal difficulty or crisis, to the best of our ability. We will not hesitate to ask each other for any specific help or support that we might want from the other of us, knowing that the help or support will be gladly and lovingly given, if possible.

Sex with others

Genital sex. As a default, a condom will be used whenever either of us shares sex involving penile penetration with another person (secondary partner). An exception may be made case by case if we agree in advance that a particular secondary partner is safe enough, in their health and personal sexual behavior (including the health and behavior of anyone with whom that person enjoys unprotected sex or has done so recently), so that condoms may be omitted.

Oral sex. Either of us may give sexual pleasure orally to another person only if we are convinced that the health risk is minimal; these decisions must be made case by case. In case of reasonable doubt, we will refrain. Since there is rather less risk of transmission from the giver to the receiver of oral sex, either of us may receive sexual pleasure orally from another person unless there is a reason to the contrary, for example, cold sores, questionable personal sex practices or history, etc.

Digital stimulation. We will refrain from digitally stimulating another person's genitals if we have any skin breaks on the hand or fingers being used for stimulation, unless a prophylactic glove is worn or a condom is used to cover a finger. We will refrain from receiving stimulation from another person digitally (without a glove or condom) if the other person has a skin break on the active hand.

Accidental exposures. In the event that a condom breaks or slips off during sex with another partner, or in the event of any other accidental exposure to bodily fluids, we will promptly inform the other of us.

Testing. Each of us will obtain complete STD testing at least once every six months as long as we are sexually involved with one or more other persons, or more often if a possible exposure renders such testing advisable.

New and renewed partners.

Introductions and agreement. Prior agreement with the other of us is not required before sharing a sexual expression of any form with a third person; we trust each other's judgment and adherence to this agreement in such matters. However, whenever practical (i.e., when a new relationship is developing and has not yet progressed to sex, but sex with the third person appears to be a possibility or likelihood), we will introduce the potential new partner to the other of us, and then subsequently (in our own privacy) we will discuss the situation between us, considering our feelings, any possible effect on our own relationship, and the degree of health risk. An introduction in person to the potential new partner is ideal, but if distance or other factors make an in-person introduction not feasible, other options (in order of preference, depending on feasibility) are introduction by telephone or introduction by computer chat or email. If none of these are feasible, we may proceed to share sex with the new partner (after screening as below), and then we will inform the other of us as soon as practical after the fact that a new sexual contact has occurred, sharing as much information as possible about the new partner and the new relationship.

Screening. Before either of us shares sex with a potential new partner, we will question the new partner carefully about their own sexual practices and ground rules, their state of health, STD testing, number of other current or recent sex partners, and any high-risk behavior that might affect the likelihood that they are an STD carrier. This inquiry will also cover any partner(s) of that person with whom unprotected sex is shared, or has been shared more recently than three months before the potential new partner's most recent testing. If we are not satisfied that the potential new partner presents an acceptably low risk, we will not share sex with that person genitally or orally, even using a condom or any other precautions. In this case, digital stimulation may be shared if attention is given to possible skin breaks, or a latex glove or condom on a finger is used.

Fluid-bonded carryover. If either of us wishes to start a new secondary sexual involvement and the potential new partner either (a) is currently sexually active or has been within six months with the other of us, or (b) is fluid-bonded with another person with whom either of us is currently sexually active or has been within six months, the screening requirement described above can be considered to be already met, unless there is information to the contrary. If either of us was sexually involved more than six months ago with the other person or with someone with whom the other person is fluid-bonded, the same principle described below under "Resumption of a suspended relationship" applies here; that is, only an updating of the other person's status is required.

Staying informed. Whenever a new ongoing secondary sexual relationship develops for either of us, we will make an agreement with the other person to communicate about any new infections or risks of infections that may occur in us, the secondary partner, or anyone with whom the secondary partner enjoys unprotected sex.

Resumption of a suspended relationship. If one of us resumes sexual involvement with someone with whom there has been no sexual sharing for more than six months, we will update the sexual hygiene information by asking the other person if there is any relevant information, such as new fluid-bonded partners or STD diagnoses, during the interim.

5.06

Communication

Knowledge of other relationships. We will each keep the other fully informed of the existence of any other developing or existing romantic and/or sexual involvements that we may have, and informed of the depth and character of each relationship and of the general nature of ongoing interactions with that person. We will also inform each other of each sexual contact with another person.

Confidentialities. Neither of us may agree with another person to hold information confidential from the other of us, although the two of us together may agree to hold another person's information confidential from others. A (temporary) exception is allowed for the specific purpose of enabling one of us to plan a gift or surprise for the other for a birthday, holiday celebration, or the like.

Communications with others. We will keep each other informed of ongoing communications between one of us and any other person with whom there is a romantic or sexual relationship or a potential new relationship, either by copying email to the other of us or by sharing the substance of any communication. This does not strictly apply to communications with friends or others with whom there is no romantic or sexual involvement, but sharing of these communications as well is encouraged. The temporary exception described above under "Confidentialities" also applies here.

~ 6 ~
Relationship Skills

Contents:
6.01. Communicate, communicate, communicate!
6.02. Styles of communication.
6.03. Dating partners for singles.
6.04. Moratorium early in your dating relationship.
6.05. Suggesting polyamory to your primary partner.
6.06. The foundation of communication among primaries.
6.07. Degrees of communication with primaries—openness and honesty.
6.08. Primaries sharing about themselves.
6.09. Sharing about your secondaries with your primaries.
6.10. Degrees of communication with secondaries.
6.11. Your children.
6.12. Keeping balance when more than two share sex (polysexuality).
6.13. Other skills, traits, and attitudes important in polyamory.

♥ ♥ ♥

6.01. Communicate, communicate, communicate!

It's a common saying in the polyamory community that there are only three basic rules that you must remember for success in polyamory: Communicate, communicate, communicate! You may also sometimes hear that referred to as the polyamory mantra.

There's a lot to be said for that bit of folk wisdom. Of course communication is also extremely important in twosome relationships, but good communication is probably *the single most* important

6.01

relationship skill when people maintain more than one emotionally and physically intimate relationship at a time, regardless of their particular variant on polyamorous relationship structure.

Knowing oneself is also right up there at the top of relationship skills important to success in polyamory, but "knowing oneself" could even be thought of as a matter of communication among various aspects of oneself, most especially between the conscious and unconscious aspects.

(Some people say that the "unconscious" aspect of the mind is misnamed, because it *is* accessible to us, becoming conscious, through certain techniques. But with that understanding, I'll continue to refer to the "unconscious mind" as the usual term for it—and it *is* unconscious, for most people.)

Most people would be amazed to discover how much of their attitudes and behavior, including their behavior toward those in the emotionally closest, most intimate relationships with them, is governed by totally unconscious aspects of their mind—mostly to the detriment of the individual and relationships. This chapter is about relationship skills of all sorts, including attitudes and nonverbal communication as well as the words that you exchange with your primary and secondary partners. And yes, psychological states like attitudes are also skills, not just traits like your height or eye color, because you can examine your attitudes for what I call "growing edges" (a term I prefer over "weak spots" or "flaws") and change and develop them as you see the need.

Hopefully, those who love you most will help point out some of these growing edges to you, as you do the same for them, but doing so in a totally loving, gentle, and supportive way of course, not criticizing or putting down. There's more on this in section 7.02 and Chapter 7 in general.

All these skills tend to blend together, so we could not have a chapter on verbal communication skills without also considering the other relationship skills.

If you are a poly-minded single person, section 6.03 deals with how you can best relate with dating partners, especially if you hope to find someone (or more than one) with whom to form a committed relationship. Later sections in this chapter will look at different areas of how, if you are now in a committed relationship, you can best communicate with your partners and relate with them lovingly and supportively.

Chapter 8 looks at communication and tactics for relating with others, such as neighbors, relatives, employers, your children's teachers, etc.

6.02. Styles of communication.

Who did what, or how you feel about it. There are several different spectra of communication to keep in mind, and failure to be aware of these differences can lead to disastrous noncommunication or miscommunication.

One spectrum involves the two basic kinds of conscious human mental activity, intellectual and emotional, or left-brained and right-brained, or mind brain and heart brain. Many people have noted a stereotypical gender difference here: Many men tend to emphasize talk about factual information (who did what when and where) while many women tend to emphasize how they feel about those things that happened, and about their associations with other people. Another spectrum, which also seems to have a gender connection, has to do with whether two people in conversation are (probably unconsciously) trying competitively to outdo the other, get "one up" on the other (the stereotypical male style), or whether (the female style) they are trying to empathize with the other, sharing and merging their awareness, supporting each other, building connections with each other.

The sociolinguist Deborah Tannen, Ph.D., in a wonderful book about these and other differences of communication styles of women and men called *You Just Don't Understand: Women and Men in Conversation* (see Appendix A for publication details), cleverly sums up men's conversation style as "report talk" and women's style as "rapport talk".

Obviously there are many individual exceptions to the gender stereotypes, and you probably have a good idea where you and your partner(s) lie on that report/rapport spectrum, regardless of the gender of each of you.

The point of it all is that everyone, and *especially* everyone who wants to lead any sort of polyamorous life successfully, regardless of their own gender or personal inclinations in this regard, needs to be aware of these usually gender-influenced innate differences of communication style, for the sake of complete left-brained and right-brained communication, and complete male-female communication, as aspects of the overall communication skills that are so important in polyamory.

Everyone in any poly relationship also needs to be quite comfortable themselves *engaging* in both "report talk" and "rapport talk" among their partners. You could think of it as a sort of bilingualism, but there is really far more involved than learning another language. (You could learn Albanian or Zulu to fluency and still be a habitual report-talker or rapport-talker.) You need to learn another way of *thinking and relating.* This is where the personal stretching may come in for you, if you are accustomed to be toward one end or the other of the report/rapport spectrum. You need to work both halves of your brain! Fill out your entire rainbow!

6.03. Dating partners for singles.

If you are single, let's suppose you meet someone interesting, the interest is mutual, so the two of you arrange a date. You "click" with each other, you have more dates, and you start doing other things together, getting to know each other pretty well, and caring for each other. Is this leading toward "forsaking all others till death do you part," or will this remain as "only" a dating relationship for the two of you, perhaps one of several relationships for each of you? Traditionally these are the only choices possible, as long as you remain truthful with each other.

But of course you know about polyamory, and so you know that a third ethical path is possible—becoming a committed primary couple but agreeing to remain open to other loving relationships that could include sex. Your dating companion may also know about polyamory, maybe not. He or she may or may not know that *you* are polyamorous.

When to mention polyamory. At what point do you bring this topic up? When you are first introducing yourself, wanting to communicate fully, you might say, "Hi, I'm Jane, and I'm polyamorous." That extreme might make you seem over-anxious to develop something deep—with *somebody, anybody, please!* The other extreme would be never to mention it unless your companion brings it up first.

The main problem with delaying that discussion, or leaving it to your companion to bring up, is that, because our mainstream culture assumes monamory (sexual exclusivity) as the "default" lifestyle, your companion is likely to assume, if you remain silent, that you're quite content to continue indefinitely with just each other (unless, of course, you met each other at a polyamory group dinner or some such), and may assume that you will "forsake all others" on your own volition, automatically, with no explicit discussion or promise necessary. It can then be quite a shock—and a potential threat to your relationship—

when you do mention your interest in polyamory down the road (maybe when you actually have in mind a potential secondary relationship with someone).

Your companion might be in a similar position, potentially interested in polyamory but holding back, embarrassed to mention it unless you bring it up first. If that happens, you both might lose out on some very nice secondary relationships just because neither of you brought up the topic of polyamory early on and it then became too "heavy" a topic for either of you to want to broach later, after the two of you had established a monamorous habit in your relationship.

Probably the best time to bring up with a dating companion the question of whether your relationship will be polyamorous is after one or a few dates (depending on how quickly things develop between the two of you). Waiting too long is not considerate of your companion, in addition to the risks mentioned above.

How to bring it up. There are a number of ways to broach the subject, and your choice of method might depend on how things seem to be developing between the two of you, as well as your own personality—how direct or indirect you like to be.

In any event, I suggest that you pick a time when you will reasonably have your companion's undivided attention for some minutes at least (in case an ongoing discussion develops, which is likely).

If your companion responds to your initial question indicating that they don't feel that the relationship has developed far enough that the two of you need to consider that question, then you don't need to press it now—and, absent an agreement to the contrary, of course you're free to date others. File the question away in the back of your mind for later—don't just ignore it indefinitely.

A direct approach. The most direct way would be simply to ask, in so many words, "I'm really enjoying dating you, and I hope we can continue. But just to prevent misunderstandings and hurt feelings down the road, how do you feel about whether or not we'll be open to dating others as well as each other, or limit ourselves just to each other?" It's always good to let others know how *you* feel about things, but eliciting your dating companion's feelings (on this or any other question) *before* offering your own is one way to show that you do care about your companion's wishes and feelings—a basic part of the respect and ethics that we consider in Chapter 3. The alternative—habitually saying "I feel like doing this" or "I'd rather have things this way," *then* finding out how your companion feels about the question, could give the impression (rightly or wrongly) that you have a tendency to be controlling or manipulative.

Of course the opposite extreme is no better. Habitually saying, "Well, what do *you* want to do?" or "Whatever you'd like, honey," without offering your own feelings, can make you seem like a chameleon or a doormat.

Your companion's response to your question about being open to dating others may launch your discussion—or you may get a rather neutral answer like "Gosh, I hadn't thought about that," or "Oh, I really don't have strong feelings one way or the other about that." If that happens, you can mention your own preference for polyamory in this relationship, and why: "Well, I *am* coming to care for you, as I think you can tell" (hand squeeze, light kiss), "but I personally feel that we could go on developing our relationship to whatever its full potential turns out to be, while we each stay open to other nice relationships that might come along. We could agree, now or later, to give our own relationship first importance, keeping any others on a secondary level. As it happens, I'm also dating one or two others right now, and I'd like to leave that option open for you too" (or) "I'm not dating anyone else right now, but I'd like to leave that option open for both of us. I know that a lot of other couples do it that way—even if they're living together or married. They keep each other informed, and keep reassuring each other that they still come first for each other. That feels right for me—so I consider myself polyamorous."

You may need to explain here what "polyamory" means (some are unclear about what's involved, even though the term is becoming better known in mainstream society), and it may be helpful for you to discuss the differences between polyamory and swinging. (See sections 1.01 and 1.02.) If your companion is interested in discussing polyamory more with you and learning more about it, you could consider giving or loaning a copy of this book, or one of the other books listed in Appendix A, section A.05.

Less direct. Perhaps you do not feel comfortable directly bringing up the question of whether your budding relationship will be polyamorous. There are things you can say to your dating companion that will indirectly reflect that you have led a polyamorous lifestyle, and would like to continue—or that you are curious about trying it, if that is the case. If your companion is alert, they may respond with questions asking details about how you prefer to relate—and so your discussion will be launched. If not, then you may decide to be more direct.

Being indirect, though, has its own pitfalls. Habitual indirectness could indicate weak self-assertiveness. Full communication requires that you share your feelings (assert yourself) as fully as is appropriate under the circumstances—and in relationships, especially polyamorous relationships, full self-assertion is very important. That's part of what is meant by that "poly mantra", "communicate, communicate, communicate."

But being indirect some of the time can be effective and healthy, as long as you communicate fully. The indirect approach for revealing your polyamorous preferences involves making casual comments (looking for opportunities to fit them into the context of conversation) about yourself or a friend that mentions having done some sort of polyamorous activity or being in a polyamorous relationship, thereby implying indirectly that you are polyamorous.

For example, "That reminds me of a time last year when my wife and I made a trip to the mountains with her secondary partner, and the three of us really enjoyed a hike that we did that day;" or, "I understand what you're saying about that politician, but I remember a time when a lover of mine invited me over to have dinner with him and his wife, and my lover said about that politician...."

When your companion asks what sort of interests and activities you're involved in (in getting acquainted with you), you can mention (along with your other activities) that you're active in your local poly social group, attending restaurant get-togethers and other group activities—or that you wish such a group existed in your area, and you'd like to help get one started. (See section 8.10 about helping to start a new local group. It's not hard.)

If you are "poly-curious", without actual poly experience, you can mention that you have learned about friends who lead a poly lifestyle; or you've read this book or seen a TV program, and it sounds interesting to you and you're curious to explore the possibilities to see if it would work well for you—for yourself or for both of you.

Your companion's response to this sort of comment could be blasé indifference, as if you'd mentioned a cousin instead of a secondary partner of yours—or your companion might respond with raised eyebrows and a question like, "What's a secondary partner?" or "Are you serious that you had a married man for a lover, who actually invited you over for *dinner* with himself and his wife? Did his wife know what was going on between you and your lover? How did *she* feel about all that?"

You could reply by explaining what a "secondary partner" is, or that your lover and his partner lead a polyamorous relationship, so that the two of them keep each other fully informed about any secondary relationships (they aren't "affairs" in the traditional sense, and neither of them is "cheating"), and everyone is comfortable with that, and you and your lover's partner are friends (maybe also lovers)—so having dinner together now and then is a natural thing to do, and everyone enjoys themself.

Now the subject of polyamory has been launched, and you can mention being inclined to polyamory yourself, as well as discussing what polyamory entails and your preferred version of it, if your new dating companion is not fully familiar with the concept and is interested in learning more.

6.04. Moratorium early in your dating relationship.

Suppose you raise the idea of polyamory to your new dating companion, as described in section 6.03, and he or she responds with something like, "Well, that idea of being open to other relationships, staying open and honest with each other about that, might work for us. But you know, since you and I are really still getting to know each other, and I really think there may be a lot of potential here between us, I'd like to focus on just you and me, at least for now. Having anyone else in either of our lives might be distracting. Besides, I find that I'm so fascinated with you that right now I just don't have any interest in dating anyone else." You may have feelings along this line yourself.

NRE. What you and your new partner are experiencing here is "new relationship energy", commonly called by its acronym, NRE, in the polyamory community. But the phenomenon certainly is not limited to polyamory; probably all new lovers experience it to some degree or another. This is the great enthusiasm and absorption early in a new love relationship in which you are all starry-eyed, and little hearts and visions of your beloved float in front of your eyes, and all you can see about your beloved is their wondrous, lovable qualities. (The dark, cobwebby corners of your beloved's personality become visible to you later, as your own cobwebs become visible to your beloved.)

The NRE phase is indeed a time for focusing on each other, learning intensely about the other person and how the two of you can mesh together in a relationship. (NRE certainly occurs as well in groups larger than two, but for simplicity of language I will assume a twosome in this following discussion.) It therefore does make sense to agree between you to limit yourselves just to each other, not dating anyone else, during this time of getting acquainted.

Sure, if you stay together for life, you will continue learning about each other to some extent indefinitely, but the early getting-acquainted process is of course most intense during the early weeks and months. It therefore makes sense to treat these first weeks and months together differently from the later phases of your relationship.

Having it both ways. If the two of you find yourselves in this situation—you hope that your relationship will develop to become primary, you want your relationship to be polyamorous, but you also want to focus on each other so you can get acquainted—you can have both by agreeing that your relationship will be polyamorous in the long term but that you will put a *moratorium* on outside (secondary) relationships for a limited time while you're developing your own relationship. The moratorium can either call for suspending all existing secondary relationships for the duration as well as not developing any new ones, or allow existing secondary relationships to continue but not allow any new ones to be started (because new relationships, whether primary or secondary, require extra time and energy in the early stages of development—the whole point of your moratorium on the primary level).

It's important to set a fixed period for the moratorium, or set a date in the future when you agree to revisit the question and decide together if you are ready yet to lift the moratorium and open your relationship to the possibility of secondary relationships. If you just say to each other, "We'll come back to this later to see if we're ready to open the relationship," without setting a specific time to do so, it may seem awkward later for either of you to broach the subject. So I suggest that the two of you agree now as to when you will revisit the question, and mark the date on both of your personal calendars (since presumably you don't have a shared calendar yet—you are not yet living together this early in your relationship).

A similar moratorium process can be used at any later point in a primary polyamorous relationship, if issues or other circumstances arise that need extra attention and energy. That is, the primary partners can agree to suspend any existing secondary relationships, or to refrain from starting any new ones, for a set period while they work on their issues or whatever the situation is. This is discussed in section 7.13.

The agreed ending date for the moratorium is not "cast in stone", of course. When the ending date comes up on the calendar, you can discuss and decide together whether to lift the moratorium or perhaps extend it a while longer.

One of you might also meet someone really attractive while the moratorium still has a ways to run. There's nothing to stop you from revisiting the moratorium agreement early, to decide whether your new primary relationship is now solid enough that you can lift the moratorium and explore the potential new secondary relationship.

6.05. *Suggesting polyamory to your primary partner.*

How to bring it up. If you are already part of a committed couple, and if you and your partner up to now have tacitly or by agreement practiced monamory, how do you suggest to your partner that you would like to open the relationship, making it polyamorous?

Do you have a skeleton in your closet? The best approach will depend on whether you have already indulged in an outside "affair" secretly, or else you have not and you would like a mutual agreement allowing each of you to have outside emotional and sexual involvements (openly and honestly) in the future. If you have already had a secret "affair" (still active or now ended) while you've been with this primary, even if it was just a one-night stand, see section 7.06. Otherwise, see the rest of this section.

Choosing a setting. Choosing a time and place for this discussion is not so critical as in the situation described in section 7.06 in which you want to come clean about a secret affair of yours. You might still prefer to find a time when you and your primary can sit for a while on your sofa without interruption from the TV or the children etc., but you could also make comments leading into this conversation at other times that happen to arise.

The difference is that if you have already had a secret "affair" (section 7.06), or violated your agreement or vows or basic ethics in some other way, you will *first* need to work with your partner to get beyond your violation of your explicit or tacit relationship agreement, and *only then* work together to build a new way of relating based on polyamory.

How to approach the subject. Rather than mentioning first that you sometimes find others emotionally or sexually attractive, or that you have someone specific in mind for yourself, I feel it would be better to come at the topic from the perspective of your shared primary relationship. There is nothing underhanded about this approach. It will be a far more positive venture if you both consider this question as an idea for broadening, enriching, and strengthening the relationship that you *share* between you, rather than seeming to search for a way of meeting the desires of *one* of you outside your primary relationship, at the possible expense of that shared relationship (or it might be seen that way to your partner). Of course, when the shared relationship is enriched, then you both also benefit individually.

With this perspective, you could suggest that your couple relationship might be broadened and enriched by expanding your friendships and involvements with other people. You could point out that mainstream society tends to restrict how close the partners in a couple may get with others, emotionally and physically, and these restrictions inevitably limit the richness of the couple relationship. But, you could point out, it's very important *to you* to avoid doing anything in *secret,* since you know that would damage the home relationship; it's important for the two members of the couple to agree on how they want to bring others into their lives. That is why you are bringing up this discussion with your partner.

Developing more friendships for both of you will probably seem self-evident. In leading into the question of whether those friendships could deepen into caring relationships that could include sex, you might want to offer your own views first this time, rather than asking first how your partner feels. Consider saying that you feel that allowing each other the freedom to develop secondary caring relationships would enrich your home relationship, rather than threatening it, as long as you both keep each other fully informed, so there aren't any secrets or surprises or unanswered questions. You could then add that, because you love your partner deeply and care about their happiness and satisfaction, you yourself would not feel threatened or jealous if your partner were to develop such a caring relationship, or express those caring feelings sexually, provided the two of you keep each other informed and have agreed in advance about the details (such as the questions discussed in Chapter 5).

If your partner responds that they feel similarly, you're on your way! (You both still have work to do, but you're on your way.)

If your partner asks you explicitly if the reason you are bringing this up is that you are interested in someone specifically, and if you are, of course you will want to answer truthfully, "yes", and give any other information asked for or that you want to volunteer (your interest's name, something about why you're interested in developing an intimate relationship with them); but you can add that you certainly want the same freedom for your partner, based on openness and honesty and mutual agreement on the details. Stress that you most certainly would not get sexually involved with this person that you're interested in behind your partner's back, in secret.

If your partner is uncomfortable. If your partner responds that they would be jealous or threatened if *you* had an outside caring connection, with or without sex, then you will certainly want to discuss this further, but this is a signal for you that your partner may have some deep-seated fears or insecurities. The two of you will need to deal with these issues first (maybe with professional help) before you can hope to establish a smoothly functioning and enriching polyamorous lifestyle.

Resolving jealousy and other forms of fear is a general psychotherapeutic problem, certainly not limited to polyamory. See section 7.05 for more about jealousy.

Your partner may agree to give polyamory a try with full enthusiasm, or with some apparent reluctance or hesitation, or with a neutral wait-and-see attitude. Especially if you seem to sense some hesitation or uncertainty in your partner about this, see section 7.12 about some possible problem areas that might surface later.

6.05

Other possible discussion threads. Let's assume for now that you do *not* run into the roadblock of jealousy. You've mentioned that what you want to talk about should enrich and strengthen your shared relationship, by opening the relationship to other caring relationships of one sort or another. You might then ask your partner about their fantasies (or review them if you already know them)—because people often feel comfortable allowing themselves to imagine scenarios as fantasies that they don't feel are possible or "right" for real life. Fantasies could include having another lover (a real person or imaginary), sharing sex with someone of the gender other than their nominal orientation, or nonstandard sexual activities like threesomes, BDSM, voyeurism and exhibitionism, fetishes, etc. Sexual fantasies could involve unlikely or impossible locations—say, in a crowded public park, on a beach, in the boss's office, on stage, on a motorcycle zooming down the highway.

You could ask your partner if they ever feel attraction to others. If you know of someone specific that your partner might be interested in, you could use that person as an example. For example: "That guy John in our hiking club seems like a nice fellow, and it seems like you and he have a lot in common. The two of you chat a lot on our hikes. Do you ever fantasize about sharing sex with him?"

Another variation would be if you observe apparent attraction toward your primary by some other person (of the appropriate gender, unless your primary is bisexual). In this case you could say something like: "You know, I get the impression that Frank might be quite interested in you. He seems to take every opportunity to hang around you, and chat with you. He does seem like a nice fellow, and you and he seem to have a lot in common. If you had the chance, would you enjoy getting to know him better, and maybe developing a sexual relationship with him?"

Your partner indicates interest in others. In the above example about John, suppose that your partner responds something like, "Mm, well, to tell the truth, John does kinda turn me on sometimes. But of course I would never do anything to hurt you or betray you. I'd never cheat on you." This is your cue to respond by letting your primary know that you would not be hurt or offended or betrayed if they did indulge in an outside relationship—provided that it was done openly and honestly, and following agreements between the two of you about sexual hygiene (Chapter 4) and in order to keep your own relationship at the highest level of importance.

Your partner indicates no interest in others. Your partner might respond to your question above with something like, "Well, John does seem like a nice guy, but my caring feelings are all for you."

Your partner might be accurately stating that they don't develop caring feelings for more than one person at a time (they are not oriented to polyamory), or it could be that they are just trying to reassure you that they have warm feelings only for you, on the *assumption* that you would be upset by learning that they found someone else attractive.

If you get this kind of response to your question, it would be helpful for you to let your partner know that you would not be bothered if your partner did develop another interest, provided (again) that the other relationship is carried out openly and honestly, and the two of you agree to give your own relationship top priority.

Having cleared up your own feelings, you may need to ask the question again, to find out whether your partner really has no inclination toward polyamory or whether they were just trying to be nice to you by hiding their feelings about the other person. If the latter, of course you need to assure your partner that you'd much rather hear their true feelings than to have those feelings shoved under the rug.

6.05

If after further discussion you learn that your partner really has no interest in poly relationships (in general, not just currently due to NRE), then you need to consider how important poly life is to you. If living polyamorously is not fundamentally important to you, you may decide to compromise away polyamorous living, so that the two of you live a monamorous relationship. Alternatively you can suggest a poly/mono relationship between you. This option is discussed further in section 2.08.

Absent real-life possibilities, asking about hypothetical lovers. If no one in real life is showing interest in your primary partner, and there is no one that your partner seems interested in, you could continue the fantasy theme, but moving it back towards the real world by asking "what if" questions, bringing up the possibility of polyamory as a theoretical possibility in your own shared life as a couple. What would your partner's feelings be if they found that they were attracted to someone else, or someone else showed interest in them? What would be your partner's feelings if *you* found yourself attracted to someone else, or someone else showed interest in you? Does your partner ever fantasize about being with someone else when the two of you are sharing sex, or at other times? Does your partner ever fantasize about being in a sexual threesome, or sharing sex with someone of the gender other than your own?

If your partner acknowledges any such fantasies or musings, you could lead this into a conversation about the fact that the two of you together, or either of you separately, can bring these fantasies to real life without hurting the relationship between the two of you, by adopting a polyamorous lifestyle, exploring the possibilities with your eyes wide open, with full openness and honesty.

If it's a totally new idea to your partner. If your partner has not previously thought much one way or the other about whether to live polyamorously, or if these concepts are totally new to them, they may not have a firm reaction one way to the other in response to the possibilities that you've raised.

If this seems to be the case (if your partner seems unsure how to respond), don't press for a definite yes-or-no immediately. Let the ideas percolate for a while. If your partner has never before seriously entertained the idea of getting sexual with anyone but you (while you've been together), or never wondered whether you might be okay with such a thing, it may take a little while for those ideas to develop (unconsciously as well as consciously). Give it some time. Your partner may bring the topic up again, or you could.

6.06. *The foundation of communication among primaries.*

Complete communication is imperative. Everyone knows that good communication is very important for any committed couple, including traditional monamorous couples. When additional relationships are added to the mix—whether secondary relationships for a polyamorous couple or additional primary relationships, creating a triad or quad, etc.—excellent communication among all primaries does not just become a good idea but becomes imperative for the success of the venture.

This section lays some groundwork that is valid for polyamorous primary dyads or for larger groups. For ease of language, in this section I will use the term "primary group" to mean either a dyad or a larger group of primaries. Chapter 9 looks at some communication and relationship dynamics that are found only in triads or larger primary groups.

Expanding one's focus from "me" to "us". So what does this deeper level of communication entail? It does not mean that absolutely everything *should* be talked about, since most of our experiences and musings and feelings are trivial and would be boring to anyone else. We mercifully drop most of that stuff from our own memories rather quickly.

It's not just a matter of *how much* to communicate; it's a matter of *focus of one's consciousness.* Is each of you in the primary group focused on what you want for yourself, or is each of you focused on the larger entity, the primary group, which consists of your partner(s) as well as yourself, and is greater than the sum of the selves?

The "barter relationship". The lowest, most primitive level of connectedness between two or more people might be called a "barter relationship". The basis of this kind of relationship is, "I'll scratch your back if you'll scratch mine. Whatever you feel your 'needs' are, I'll try to meet them for you, provided you do the same for me." (I put "needs" in quotes because when the vast majority of people talk about "getting their needs met", they are really referring to *wants,* not real needs. There's nothing wrong with *wanting* things for oneself, but let's be clear on just how essential they are or are not.)

The problem with this rather mercantile attitude as a basis for personal relationships is that if I decide my back has been scratched enough and no longer itches, I'm inclined to shift my attention away from scratching yours. The barter breaks down. There is really no group energy here, just separate individuals wandering around the bazaar, each looking to satisfy their own individual desires, and they want some help doing so. There is nothing inherently wrong with this, but people often never notice the very self-oriented nature of this kind of relationship, nor do they discover that a great deal more is possible in personal interrelationships, by widening their outlook from "me" to "us"—and then from "both of us" to "all of us".

Modifying the Golden Rule. The Golden Rule, in its standard wording that we are familiar with in western cultures, wonderful as it is, does not quite promote barter relationships, but it comes so close that it is easy to see how people could take it that way without even being aware that they are doing so.

That standard wording in English says, "Do unto others as you would have them do unto you." Look at the wording closely and you will see that it is really self-centered. It advises us to treat everyone else according to *our own* preferences and tastes, rather than what *the other person* might prefer. It does not recognize that the other person's preferences might differ from our own.

If you like science fiction, the Golden Rule would urge you to buy a science fiction novel as a gift for your friend's birthday, even if your friend has no interest in science fiction. If your inclination happens to be to do your own thing and you don't care much whether you get praise or criticism or no comment at all on what you do (a valid preference), you may tend not to give your partner much feedback, even though your opinions and comments may be much more important to them than theirs are to you. If this happens, your partner is likely to form the opinion that you are aloof, distant, and uncaring, while you may come to feel that your partner is meddlesome and demanding.

If you're horny and single, you will look for someone who meets your description of the kind of person you'd enjoy sharing sex with (scratching each other's itch). If you find such a person, and that person feels similarly about you, you may say (and even sincerely believe), "Oh, you're so attractive and sexy! I love you!" This person "scratches your itch," and you scratch theirs. The catch, again, is that this is still self-centered. "Attractiveness" is not really an objective quality of the other person; it's that someone whom *you are attracted to* meets *your* (current) desires (or you feel that they could).

The author Tony Alessandra, Ph.D., has also noted the self-centered nature of the Golden Rule, and has proposed a slight modification to it, which he calls the "Platinum Rule" (and he holds a trademark on that

6.06

phrase). The "Platinum Rule" says: *Do unto others as they would have you do unto them.* Dr. Alessandra has written a number of books on the subject, and he offers seminars, etc., mostly from the perspective of business rather than personal psychology. (See Appendix A.) But the principle is certainly equally valid for interpersonal relationships.

By shifting from the Golden Rule to the Platinum Rule, now we are focused on the other person and their wishes, and on our relationship with them, rather than on our own desires first and foremost. The focus of our attention has been ratcheted up one level. Instead of being two atomic individuals, now we are a molecular dyad.

Of course part of what it means to be a molecule that follows the Platinum Rule is that that other atom over there on the other side of this molecule is also doing unto you according to what *you* want, not according to its own odd quirks. Everything should balance out.

At first glance this may seem not very different from what I called a "barter relationship", but in fact it is diametrically different. The "barter relationship" is self-centered; the new relationship, based on the Platinum Rule, is centered on your partner(s) and on the partnership, while your partner(s) are centered on you and on their partnership with you—and that in turn generates an energy, a bond, a stability, among you.

I spoke of ratcheting up our attention or our consciousness. This phenomenon does not have to stop there. Now our consciousness has ratcheted up from our own atomic self to the molecular level of a couple or small primary group. When our couple or small group finds itself interrelating with other similar couples or groups, and since we are thinking now on that group level and applying our modified Golden Rule yet again, we ratchet our consciousness up one more level, to groups on the next larger size level.

And so on. And through it all, our individual desires will also get satisfied, because they are in harmony with those of the larger groups.

Do you begin to see now what might be possible through polyamory? Of course these sorts of ideas are nothing new; bodhisattvas and sages and shamans in all human cultures have been trying in various ways for many thousands of years to tell us about the Universal Consciousness of which we are each an atom or a cell (choose your metaphor).

This is not meant to be a somber, "preachy" sort of commentary. As for myself, I feel that the prospects of expanding my level of consciousness more and more broadly should be lots of fun.

6.07. Degrees of communication with primaries—openness and honesty.

The phrase "openness and honesty", heard in polyamory circles even more than "communicate, communicate, communicate," is usually taken to mean keeping your primary partner(s) thoroughly informed about your secondary relationships. "Multiple emotional and sexual involvements are okay as long as they're done openly and honestly—no lying or secrecy—and everyone is okay with it."

The phrase certainly does include that meaning, but (as with so much else in polyamory) it really has a more far-reaching meaning, including a far more complete degree of sharing of information and inner feelings between primary partners, and keeping secondary partners reasonably well in the picture as well.

It's a degree of personal sharing to which many, probably most, people are unaccustomed, even those who typically do share their feelings with others easily. Being more forthcoming and expressive about your inner thoughts and feelings to those who are closest to you can only be good, so your development, and your partners' development, of these

6.07

behavior skills and habits can be nothing but positive and growthful for each of you.

Beyond that broad description of "openness and honesty", different degrees of communication with both primaries and secondaries may be appropriate or desired.

"Don't ask, don't tell." The bare minimum for a functionally possible level of "openness and honesty" would seem to be the "don't ask, don't tell" arrangement, whereby a couple agree that either may have outside sexual relationships, but they agree not to offer nor ask for any information at all even as to whether any such secondary relationships exist, much less identity or any other details.

This may work if both agree to it, but it is awkward, because each partner has to concoct cover stories, as much as for a secret "affair", for blocks of time when they are with a secondary. Beyond that, the stated desire by one partner not to know details raises serious questions about how comfortable that person really is with polyamory in general. They may agree to or suggest the "don't ask, don't tell" arrangement out of a well-meaning desire to compromise, and to honor their partner's desire for polyamory, but their agreement may be grudging, reflected by their desire not to know anything further beyond the fact that their partner *may* have a secondary relationship active at any point.

If this is the case for you and your partner, you may wish to consider trying a "poly/mono" arrangement instead of "don't ask, don't tell". This poly/mono arrangement can work well when one partner wants a poly relationship and the other does not but accepts that the first partner may have outside relationships, with whatever agreements they may make about safe sex, sharing of details, etc. Poly/mono relationships are discussed more fully in section 2.08. See Chapter 5 about the relationship agreement.

Intermediate levels of communication. A wide range of degree of factual disclosure between primary partners is possible within the general principle of "open and honest", between "don't ask, don't tell" at one extreme and the other extreme of copying all email and online chats and describing all voice conversations and personal interactions. Some primaries like to know that a secondary relationship exists and with whom (name shared), and that's enough. Some want to be introduced in person to a potential new secondary partner before that new relationship becomes sexual, or promptly afterwards—and then they don't care whether or not there is further interaction. Some like to develop at least a nonsexual friendship with their primary's secondary, and some (if the sexual orientations allow it) like to develop a sexual relationship themselves with anyone with whom their primary is sexual. As with so much else in polyamory, the variations are infinite.

6.08. Primaries sharing about themselves.

We noted in section 6.01 that good communication skills are very important in monamorous couple relationships but are imperative for a polyamorous couple or a larger primary group. This section will look at how sharing information and feelings on a level deeper than most couples are probably used to can strengthen your primary relationship and improve your overall experience with polyamory—even though some of the information and feelings revealed may not be very pretty.

Getting acquainted. In the early stages of a relationship, as you are getting to know each other, you learn basics about each other, such as age, whether you're now in a committed relationship, whether you have children, what your interests and recreations are, your philosophical and spiritual views, your tastes in music, how you earn your living, and such.

6.08

Getting stuck. Many couples never go much beyond these superficial basics—plus maybe things like learning how dark their partner likes their toast, whether they take cream in their coffee, and which way they like to put the toilet paper into the holder. A monamorous couple can often base a "successful" relationship on information about each other that is not much deeper than this—"successful" in the sense that they manage not to separate.

Perhaps you have known people who have been married 10, 30, 50 or more years who seem to fit this category. Perhaps you see someone like that in the mirror. If the latter is the case, do not despair. Relationships that have gone dormant, or maybe never really "woke up" beyond those basics, can be energized and vitalized, often. That said, I don't think anyone would claim that *every* moribund or shallow or dysfunctional relationship can be salvaged or raised above its current minimal level.

Let's suppose, though, that either you're in a relationship in which getting to know each other is still a fairly fresh thing; or you and your partner have gotten into some ruts but you both would like to get back to the exciting NRE of your early relationship, and maybe pick up where you left off and move on to still greater heights. (Hurrah for you both!) Or maybe you're now unattached—maybe having come out of a relationship that died for lack of binding energy—and you'd like to know in advance how to proceed better next time.

Beyond the basics. Don't stop with learning age, likes and dislikes, and which way you each like the toilet paper to come off the roll. Share with your partner in depth what you were like as a child, and what your birth family was like. As we all know, childhood experiences and impressions do have a profound effect on the rest of one's life. Sometimes we consciously or unconsciously stay in the same mold into which we were kneaded as a child. Sometimes we consciously decide in adolescence or adulthood that we don't like something about how we were shaped in childhood and we work to make ourselves different. Our own quirks may therefore closely resemble those of one or both of our parents—or by conscious effort we may have become very different indeed from our parents. Let your partner know which is the case for you.

Either way, telling your partner about your childhood, including most especially your *feelings about* your childhood, and listening about your partner's, can enormously strengthen your understanding of each other's inner workings and thereby strengthen the bond between you. When your bond is stronger, you will both be in a much better position to enjoy the delights of one or more secondary relationships without feeling a threat to your primary relationship.

It isn't all pretty. What you learn about each other won't all be sweetness and light and spring flowers. You will learn about each other's "growing edges" (weak spots) as well as strengths. This is a good thing. If you are much better at something than your partner, this does not need to become a wedge working to divide you. You can be a team, with each of you doing what you're better at. If you're better at something than your partner is, help them (lovingly, supportively)—and graciously accept their help with your own "growing edges".

See section 7.04 about "hot buttons". You may encounter some of these "hot buttons" in your partner, and your partner may come across some in yourself, during the process of getting acquainted described above.

Make it a habit. Probing each other's psyches in this loving way, and opening ourselves to our partner's probing, should become a habit between you. We all (some more than others) have a tendency to keep the doors shut on the dark, cobwebby recesses of our own minds and histories—and we all have those cobwebby recesses. We also tend not to ask questions that would peer too closely into those cobwebby recesses of those we love most, out of a concern not to cause them discomfort. But if each of you has gotten used to opening those doors in yourself, without shame or embarrassment, as we carry forward the process of *really* getting to know ourselves and each other, then it will be easier for each of you to swing your own doors wide for your partner(s), on an ongoing basis. Not just your polyamorous involvements but all aspects of your lives will be much the richer for it.

As noted earlier, you may be well along in a relationship, and now you feel you've fallen into ruts; you learned something about each other early on, then you closed your own doors and you stopped asking to see behind your partner's doors. Don't let that stop you from trying now what I've described above. For you it'll involve a change in habits, but we all know that habits *can* be changed. You can take it slow and easy with each other. But each of you can expect to find great rewards, as you each reactivate and deepen the process of getting acquainted. Persevere with this.

6.09. Sharing about your secondaries with your primaries.

Information about your secondaries. As you and your primary partner(s) discuss how much detail of information you each want to know about the other's secondaries, keep in mind that anything that is unknown tends to loom larger than real life in the imagination, especially if it is perceived as negative or threatening, or if there is any potential of such a perception. The more information you give your primary(-ies) about your secondaries and what you do with them, the less likely (all else being equal) your primary(-ies) will be to wonder if the other person might become a threat to the primary relationship.

Who? If you have become interested in someone new, what is this person's name? Gender? Sexual orientation? Approximate age? How did you meet? Where do they live (how far away)? What are they like as a person (personality, recreations and other interests, likes and dislikes, strengths and weaknesses, philosophy, spiritual understanding, profession)? (Some of these things, of course, will take a while to learn.) Why are you interested in dating this person or getting to know them better? Physical description? Is this person in a committed relationship or unattached? If in a relationship, is that relationship polyamorous? (Is this person's spouse or partner aware of the interest between this person and you, or would it be a secret "affair" if it develops?) How careful are this person's general habits of sexual hygiene with other sex partners of theirs? Have they had recent STD testing? (How big a health risk do they present, even with condom use?)

Introduce each other? Would your primary partner(s) like to meet your new interest in person, perhaps before you become further involved with them? Would an introduction by phone, online chat, or email suffice? Might your primary(-ies) possibly be interested in developing a relationship of their own with this new interest, and vice versa? This could range anywhere from a fairly casual platonic friendship, through a secondary-level sexual involvement, up to becoming a new primary partner in a triad (or whatever your current primary group size is, plus one). If your new interest is also in a committed relationship, would you, your primary(-ies), your new interest, or their primary(-ies), want to meet each other, with all of the same above possibilities?

What, where, when. If you have already had a date with your new interest, when was it? What did you do and where did you go with that person on your date? What did you talk about? Did you share sex? What kind of sex (oral, genital, anal)? Was it threesome or moresome sex? Did you use a condom? What sorts of sexual expression does your new friend enjoy? Did you stay overnight together? Did you make plans to see each other again? Would you like to, or do you feel it was a dead-end after one date?

6.09

Rehearse in advance. It can be helpful for you and your primary(-ies) to consider how you would answer questions such as those above about a *hypothetical* new interest, before an actual situation arises—before one of you actually meets someone and you find yourself in the position of saying, "By the way, honey, I've met someone really interesting, and we want to meet for dinner sometime soon and get better acquainted."

Sit down together with your primary and discuss how you each feel, while it's still hypothetical. This way you can take as much time as you'd like for pondering different alternatives, including multiple discussion sessions if desired. You may wish to include some of your decisions in your relationship agreement (Chapter 5). Then when a real situation arises—one of you really does meet someone interesting—it should go far more smoothly and efficiently. Of course you and your primary partner(s) may want to modify your agreements on these questions based on your real-life feelings *after* one of you has a date with someone else or starts a real-life secondary relationship.

If there's already someone out there. If you are already interested in someone, and you have not previously talked in hypothetical terms as described above (but assuming you do at least have an agreement to live polyamorously), then let your partner(s) know that you have a potential new interest, and assure your partner(s) first off that you will proceed with this new person, or not, based on what you and your primary partner(s) decide, after you've had a chance to talk about it together.

If you and your partner have not yet agreed to live polyamorously but you would like to (so you can develop a secondary relationship with this new person openly and honestly), see section 6.05.

If you and your partner have not yet agreed to live polyamorously but you have already become sexually involved with someone else in secret from your partner, there are ethical implications, and your situation is delicate. If this is your situation, see sections 7.06 through 7.10.

Keep your partner(s) up to date about your feelings about your secondary. Always letting your primary partner(s) know about your secondary partner and what you do with your secondary is clearly important—but it is even more important to keep your primary(-ies) thoroughly informed about your *feelings* about your secondary partner or that relationship. This is especially important in the early phases of a new secondary relationship, but it is important as well as the secondary relationship evolves and matures. Is this someone you enjoy being with, maybe taking to bed, but that's about all? Do you find your affection for this person growing into a strong fondness? Love? Do you find yourself entertaining the notion that you might like to bring this person into your existing primary relationship as a new primary partner? Or, as time passes, do your feelings for the other person more or less level off, or maybe start to wane?

Be sure to keep your primary partner(s) up to date about your feelings about this secondary relationship as time passes.

6.10. Degrees of communication with secondaries.

Previous sections make it clear how important it is to have thorough, deep communication among primaries, although there is some room for personal preferences. The situation is somewhat different with regard to secondary relationships, simply because the depth or intensity of these relationships can vary so much, from quite casual "friend with benefits" relationships up to very deep and strongly loving and long-lasting relationships that resemble primary relationships in many respects.

In the mainstream world, someone who dates more than one person at a time may feel no obligation to share with one dating partner even the fact that there are other dating relationships, although ethically anyone should reveal if they are already in a *committed* relationship (marriage or comparable). The general practice in polyamory is for greater disclosure to secondaries.

Even with a very casual dating relationship, in polyamory, a minimum of respect would suggest letting the person know if you are in a committed relationship and whether you have other dating relationships. Beyond that, there are fewer ethical or practical reasons to share deeply with a secondary in the ways that I suggest in the preceding sections than there are for sharing deeply and thoroughly with a primary—but I still feel that there are the same potential benefits and rewards for sharing more deeply with a secondary as there are with a primary. It's just that with a secondary the stakes are perhaps not as high. Even so, by sharing more deeply with a secondary, you are likely to find that the secondary relationship is strengthened and enriched. So my bottom line on this question is, the more sharing of information and feelings with a secondary, the better.

6.11. *Your children.*

It's well known that young children will not learn things presented to them before they're developmentally capable of grasping the concepts. (Come to think of it, the same might be said of humans of any age—but we're talking about kids here.) On the other hand, children are extremely good observers and will generally learn better by what they see and hear around them than by being told a string of words.

Furthermore, if there is a conflict between what a child is told and what they observe, they will take to heart what they observe. (Again, this is no different for adults.) A child will consider that their parents, teachers, or others in their lives are hypocrites if the latter's deeds do not match their words—for example, if parents lecture their children to keep their rooms neat, but the parents leave the rest of the house messy, toss cigarette butts and other litter on the ground, etc., or if a teacher asks the students to be polite to each other but then behaves rudely toward the students.

I once saw a touching family scene of a man out bicycling with his daughter, who appeared to be about six years old. The little girl was dutifully wearing a helmet—but Daddy had no helmet. What was that little girl learning?

Telling children about your polyamorous life. So do you tell your children that you are polyamorous? In how much detail? When? How?

A couple with children. If you try to hide your polyamorous involvements from your children, you are in a difficult situation similar to trying to maintain a "don't ask, don't tell" policy with your primary partner. How do you explain to your children when you are away from home with a secondary, or a secondary visits your home, or you spend time on the phone or in online chat with a secondary? If you invent "white lies" to cover these situations, your children will sooner or later realize that you are hiding things from them and not telling them the truth—and from then on they will think of you as prone to lying, and not trustworthy about what you say in general.

There are several reasons why your children should be told the truth, or as much of the truth as they are capable of understanding at their level of maturity. Building and maintaining your reputation with them as a truth-teller is one fundamental reason. Another reason is that your children may hear remarks from others who have seen or heard things. If your children have no idea that you date others, then they may consider these remarks from others to be an unjustified smear campaign against you. If you have tried to hide your polyamorous activities from your children but they have suspected and concluded that you've lied to them and kept secrets, then remarks from others will put them in an even more difficult position. They are likely to conclude

6.11

that you are doing something mysterious and bad of which you are too ashamed to let them know. Of course this sets a very bad example for your children.

It is better, then, I feel, to let your children know that you and your partner have "special friends" that you like to spend time with. If your children are pre-puberty, you can leave it at that, since they probably will not understand romance and sex. If they have passed puberty and understand these things, I feel it is best to let them know that you and your partner share sex with your "special friends", because the children will wonder and suspect it even if you say nothing about that. (You could include this information into your conversations with them about sex education.)

But it is also appropriate to point out to your children that information about your sexual involvements with others is personal information that they should keep to themselves unless you let them know otherwise, because telling others would not be fair to the other person's privacy. You can point out that you and your partner don't spread this information freely either (if that's the case).

As your children grow into adolescence and come to understand romantic relationships, it would also be good to have a talk with them at some point about what polyamory is and the fact that you and your partner (or just one of you if it's poly/mono) follow this lifestyle, proudly and ethically. If you and your partner try to remain "in the closet", of course you will need to explain the "closet" to your children and why you and your partner feel the need to stay in it. Obviously this aspect is easier if you are "out of the closet".

A triad or larger group with children. When children grow up in a household with three or more partners, it will become obvious to the children at a fairly early age that their family is different from most, because most of their school friends have a mommy and a daddy, or one or the other if there's been a separation or death. So who is this third or fourth adult who lives with us? When a child is still rather young (pre-puberty), it should be enough to explain that all the adults who live here at home love each other a lot, and so we all want to live together. As the children pass puberty and come to understand romance and sex, they can also understand that various combinations among the adults at home enjoy a sexual involvement with each other, as an expression of their mutual love.

Obviously a triad or larger group that lives together cannot be "in the closet" about their own relationship, although hypothetically they could keep secret the fact that they also have secondary relationships, if they do. If there are contacts with secondaries, this can be explained to the children as in the case of a poly couple as described above.

6.12. Keeping balance when more than two share sex (polysexuality).

When three or more people enjoy sex together, it's called "polysexuality".

There are a number of possible combinations and variations here, but one concern is common to all permutations. Let's say you're in a couple, and you (A) or your partner (B), or both of you together, develop a sexual interest with someone else (C). If A, B, and C are all hetero, then a sexual "V" will be created (see section 2.04), and C will share sex with either A or B, depending on C's gender. If both people of the same gender are bi, then adding C can create a sexual triangle. There are other permutations if one or more of these three are gay or lesbian.

Or, a couple Z and A may meet and want to share sex together with another couple, Y and B. Similar permutations are possible as with a threesome, only more so.

Because the same problem can occur in any of these combinations, let's look at the simple case of two hetero couples Z-A and Y-B. As we've done in earlier sections, let's say that Z and Y are male, A and B are female. You arrange a date, you all "click" together, and in time all four of you are in bed together—or maybe sprawled in the living room or cozying up in the hot tub.

You will most probably want to focus on the new combinations—Z with B, A with Y. But what if A and B (the two women) both start focusing their attention on one of the guys—Z or Y? Or if Z and Y start focusing on one of the women? Someone is going to feel left out, unless one of the four happens to enjoy watching (being a voyeur). This situation happened to my primary and me once. It shut things down really fast!

When there are four in bed together, clearly threesome combinations are also possible along with two pairs. But it is far better to put off exploring these threesome possibilities right at first, to prevent anyone from feeling left out, unless one of you does enjoy watching. You can pair off, or else have a foursome "group grope". After you have all enjoyed each other in this way, being sure that all four are included, then if you wish to get together further, you can try the four different threesome combinations at different times if you want, leaving one of you at a time on the sidelines as spectator and cheerleader.

6.13. Other skills, traits, and attitudes important in polyamory.

Most of these skills, traits, and attitudes are important and valuable in monamorous dyadic relationships; they are even more important or imperative in polyamory.

Trust. When your primary partner is heading off on a date with a new love interest, with your knowledge and blessing, perhaps the most essential and fundamental quality for *you* to maintain at this time is trust in your partner—trust that they will honor their love for you and their commitment to you, not diminishing you in their heart at the same time that they may be building someone new up in their heart. Trust is surely one of the most fundamental attitudes serving as the foundation for success in living polyamorously.

Trust does not come automatically nor as something that we just decide to do. We cannot say to our partner, "Okay, let's agree to trust each other, since we can each have our secondary relationships that way;" or, "Even though I've lied to you or betrayed you before, I'm asking you to start trusting me now so that I can develop a secondary relationship."

Trust must be *earned and developed.* Before A can trust B, B has to *demonstrate* to A that B is trust*worthy*. A has to learn enough about B's character to become confident that B is honest, honorable, ethical; that B will honor their commitments, always tell the truth, and take another person's feelings into consideration, not seeking solely to fulfill their own personal desires. When A has come to know B well enough, and if the notion of some possible deception or betrayal then comes to mind, A will then be able to say with full confidence, "No, B would never do that." That's trust.

Trust is also very fragile. If B does indeed do something contrary to the relationship of trust that has been carefully cultivated, even only once, the trust will be seriously damaged, possibly destroyed. It may never be possible to restore it; or, at best, it can be restored only after much work by both parties—by B to try to reassure A of B's trustworthiness; by A to become convinced that there won't be another betrayal.

This dynamic is why "cheating" is taken so seriously in the mainstream world—and rightly so. There is a tacit or explicit agreement

6.13

by both partners in a mainstream couple never to share sex with anyone else. If one partner does so, it is not the outside sex itself that causes the problem; rather, the other partner's *trust* in the offending partner is damaged or shattered, with obvious serious consequences for the relationship.

"Cheating" is certainly also possible among polyamorous partners, although the word "cheat" is not heard as much in the poly community as in the mainstream. "Cheating" in polyamory would consist of violating the terms of your relationship agreement—and polys would probably word it in terms of a "violation of our agreement".

Several sections in Chapter 3 deal with this dynamic in more depth.

Self-esteem and self-confidence. Jealousy results from fear, primarily fear that your partner's interest in or involvement with someone else may escalate to pull your partner away from you. The new person (so you fear) may be more physically or emotionally attractive, more exciting than yourself in sex, or better in any of a number of imagined ways.

An excellent antidote or preventive for jealousy therefore is to have a good self-esteem, so you are confident that you can be as good a partner, in bed or otherwise, as anyone else.

Of course life has no guarantees. You might lose your partner even if your partner never develops a relationship with anyone else (witness the divorce rate among the mainstream population). But good self-esteem is high among the personal qualities that maximize your chances of keeping your partner happily committed to you.

With self-esteem you accept the possibility of losing your primary partner as one of life's inevitable risks, hopefully a small risk. Your sense of self is *inside yourself,* not projected onto your partner, and so you know that even if the worst-case scenario occurs and your partner decides to leave you, you still have yourself at least, and your odds of finding someone new will be good (though if there *is* a separation you probably will not want to jump back into the dating scene immediately—it is better to go through a grieving period for a lost relationship).

Self-assertiveness. Because polyamorous dynamics are complicated, you will need to be especially alert to express your wishes and your preferences to your primary partner(s). In a dyad it may be possible (although not healthy) to hang back and let your partner make the decisions with little input from you. In a polyamorous relationship this is both more difficult and more likely to lead to problems. So stick up for yourself (nicely) and keep your primary relationship egalitarian. If you enjoy dom-sub games, keep them on the level of games, not real life.

Empathy. Section 6.06 speaks of expanding your consciousness from "me" to "us". If you do this you will need to be constantly alert to what your partner(s) are feeling, or may be feeling even if they don't express it. If any doubt, ask. Then take your partner's feelings into account. How would they likely react if I did such-and-such with my secondary? With practice this can become more accurate and second-nature.

Compersion. An equivalent term in some English-speaking countries is "frubble".

Sometimes called the opposite of jealousy, compersion can be described as feeling joy when your primary partner (or anyone you love) shares loving feelings or activities with someone else—because your love for your partner means that you genuinely want your partner to have a joyous, rich life. Your partner is in your life not just for your own self-gratification—not just to scratch *your* itch (as in the "barter relationship"—section 6.06).

Compersion is thus a type of empathy. Also see the entry for "compersion" in the Glossary (Appendix B). If you have a tendency toward jealous feelings when your love shows interest in someone else (maybe it's a "hot button" for you—see sections 6.09 and 7.04), it may take some introspection and practice and support from your partner(s) for you to grow beyond your habitual feelings so that you feel compersive joy for your partner.

Flexibility. Polyamorists are fond of pointing out that although love may be infinite, there are only 24 hours in a day, 7 days in a week. Scheduling among multiple loving partners can be a challenge. Plans sometimes have to be changed, or put off farther into the future than you would like because the calendar is already so full. For planning things both with your primary partner(s) and with your secondaries, it helps to be accepting of the occasional need to reschedule or put things off. You can also be flexible about where you go and what you do or where you are at a given time, to more smoothly accommodate your dates with your secondaries, your activities with your primary(-ies), and your primary's dates with their secondaries. Section 8.02 discusses scheduling in detail.

Compromise. There are so many possible variations in polyamory that it is very likely that you and your primary partner(s) will run up against at least some differences of preferences on how to conduct your primary relationship. Stand up for what you feel strongly (see "Self-esteem" above in this section), but you and your partner(s) should be willing to compromise when a difference arises and each of you can comfortably live with something other than your first preference.

Being willing to stand out in the crowd. If you want to live polyamorously, you could choose to remain "in the closet", but as long as mainstream culture considers polyamory to be on the fringe or worse, those who are willing to let their polyamory be publicly visible will be doing a service for themselves and future polyamorists (and indeed for society as a whole) by helping those in the mainstream come to see

6.13

polyamory as one of several acceptable and ethical forms for people to relate with the ones they love.

"Standing out in the crowd" can be something as simple as three people hugging or walking hand-in-hand-in-hand in a public place such as a sidewalk or a park; it can be making direct or indirect allusions to your multiple love relationships in conversation and mail with friends, relatives, coworkers, and others in the mainstream. More proactively, "standing out" can also involve being a political activist for establishing or preserving basic civil rights for polyamorists, lobbying for new legislation, going to court to pursue rights or to challenge bigotry or discrimination, etc. Section 8.11 discusses political activism more fully.

~ 7 ~
Resolving Issues

Contents:
7.01. Overview.
7.02. Qualities to bring to the table.
7.03. Heal old stuff first.
7.04. "Hot buttons".
7.05. Jealousy.
7.06. If you've "cheated" in a monamorous relationship—preparations.
7.07. The actual discussion—coming clean about the past.
7.08. Continuing the discussion—looking to the future.
7.09. Continuing the discussion—if your partner also confesses to "infidelity".
7.10. If the "affair" was your partner's in a monamorous relationship.
7.11. Violations of a polyamorous relationship agreement.
7.12. Hidden psychological resistance.
7.13. Moratoriums.
7.14. Professional counseling or healing help.
7.15. Polyamory support groups.
7.16. Growing out of a relationship.

♥ ♥ ♥

7.01. Overview.

Resolve, don't ignore. What follows here will sound like another variation on a theme that has already appeared more than once in previous chapters. Conflict resolution, not shoving problems under the

7.01

rug, is very important in traditional monamorous relationships—but in polyamory it becomes at the same time much more important and much more complex. It is more important because a solid consensus or common outlook is more important as a basis of any relationship involving more than two people. It is more complex because the issues among more than two people tend to involve more possible variations, ramifications, dimensions.

For this reason it is imperative for you, if you wish to live polyamorously, to develop good skills for conflict resolution and also to be ready and willing to engage in the conflict resolution process with your partner(s). Conflict resolution requires neither submissively yielding to your partners' positions in the misguided expectation of preserving domestic tranquility nor stubbornly, unyieldingly hanging onto your pet views and attitudes when your partner(s) are lovingly suggesting an alternative for your consideration.

People speak of "winning" or "losing" an argument. Arguing will *not resolve* conflicts, because conflict resolution is not a competition, where one person's view "wins" and the other "loses". When a conflict has been resolved, all parties have found a common ground together that they can agree about and be happy about.

Section 9.11 points out that when the two people in a dyad come upon a disagreement, they may make a good-faith effort to resolve it, but they may end up simply "agreeing to disagree". Of course this may happen in a triad or larger group as well, but for the multi-adult group it is more important to search diligently for a resolution, so that "agreeing to disagree" would really be a last resort. The search for resolution is also more important for a polyamorous dyad (with secondary relationships) than for a monamorous dyad. Poly life is simply more involved, and an unresolved conflict has more potential for boat-rocking.

So if a disagreement comes up among you, don't let it linger. Sit down together and do your best to resolve it, using the best that is in each of you (see section 7.02) and using the techniques discussed in this chapter (and Chapter 9 if you are in a triad or larger group), and any other assets that you have available.

Do not hesitate to seek professional counseling if the problem seems to defy resolution on your own (see section 7.14), or take your issue to a local poly support group if available (section 7.15).

Chapter 9 looks at the dynamics that are special in triads and larger primary groups, including techniques for conflict resolution in those groups larger than two.

Other resources. There are many books, many seminars and workshops, and other resources available that are designed to help committed *couples* understand and resolve their misunderstandings and disagreements, develop techniques for interrelating smoothly and lovingly, and raise their general level of relating to a higher level. Generally speaking, these resources work just as well when more than two people are involved, because the same basic psychological processes are in action. I therefore strongly recommend that you avail yourselves of these resources.

See Appendix A for recommended books and resources.

7.02. Qualities to bring to the table.

Pick a good time and place. As section 7.06 describes for the particularly thorny situation of coming clean to your partner about having broken an agreement of sexual exclusivity, having a good setting for a discussion about any issue or disagreement is important. Don't launch into a complaint about your partner, or confess to a misdeed, when you're standing in the check-out line at the grocery store or when one of you is about to head out the door to work. When your partner first walks in the door after work is not a good time either! Give them a chance to kick off their shoes and relax a bit!

Look for a time when both or all of you will be able to devote a chunk of time to the discussion, without interruptions. You may want to suggest a time in advance. This has the added advantage of preventing your partner(s) from feeling that you're springing something on them suddenly, as they might feel if you just launch into your comments (no matter how well presented) without warning. So, you might say something like, "Say, honey, I have something that I'd to talk about with you. It shouldn't be a big problem, but if we can sort through it together, that might help our relationship be just a little smoother. Would this evening after dinner" (or) "this evening after the kids have been put to bed be a good time to sit on the sofa and talk for a few minutes?"

This may seem self-evident, but when you do sit down to talk, be sure the TV is off. Gentle music can be nice—nothing loud, jarring, or distracting, and nothing vocal, because words draw attention to themselves. It is better to use your own recordings than to have the radio playing, to avoid occasional verbal interruptions by the announcer.

Bring the right attitudes. When you and your primary partner(s) sit down to discuss a disagreement or issue, it is important that each of you *not* come to the figurative "table" with the attitude of trying to defend your position, or of trying to "win" a competition with your partners. This is not a court proceeding, and it is not a debate or contest or competition. Your ego is not at stake here. The goal is to find common ground, and you'll all be the happier when you find it. (Speaking of ego, no doubt your ego will feel that it is much better off when it can take pride in succeeding at resolving the current issue along with that really nice ego in that other body sitting next to you.)

Even if you approach the discussion with this goal of seeking common ground, what if your partner jumps into a competitive stance, seemingly trying to "win an argument" over you? If it looks like this might be the case, first, resist the natural temptation to fall into arguing back. If you do, you both will have lost already. Rather than giving a retort even if it's responsive to your partner's argumentative question, pause a moment, then say calmly that you'd like for the discussion to be about seeking common ground where you both can win, along the lines of the paragraph above.

Section 6.13 lists several general qualities or attitudes that I feel are important to cultivate in oneself for success and happiness in all aspects of living polyamorously. Those qualities and attitudes are probably most important when you and your partner(s) come upon an issue that needs resolution, so I'll just mention them again here: trust; self-esteem and self-confidence; respectful self-assertiveness; empathy; compersion; flexibility; compromise. There is some commentary on each of those in section 6.13.

Stay alert for nonverbal signals. A very high percentage of interpersonal communication, especially about emotional states, takes place without words—things like facial expressions, grunts and mumbles, body stance, pauses before answering a question, tone of voice, word choice, fumbling for words more than usual, choice of emotionally loaded words rather than less charged synonyms, periods of silence, interruptions, and the like.

There is a natural tendency, even when we notice these nonverbal expressions, not to focus on them. However, especially in poly relationships, we ignore these signals at our peril. I'm not suggesting that we should pick fights with our partners, but when we notice some gesture or tone of voice in our partner that suggests that the other person is annoyed, or jealous, or tired, or hurt, it's a very good idea to ask them about it explicitly. "Honey, is something bothering you?" "Did I say something to hurt you?" The response may be, "No, I'm just tired," or "No, I just have a bit of a headache." Or, you may get, "Well, yeah, and thanks for asking. I couldn't help but notice how you seemed really fascinated with that other guy/gal at our poly group gathering this evening. I felt sorta left out."

Now that your partner has put their feelings into words, you can take it from there, express your own feelings, and bring things back to an even keel; then deal with the substantive issue at hand.

7.03. *Heal old stuff first.*

As the partners in a poly dyad or larger primary group undergo personal growth, inevitably they will gain insights into old dysfunctional psychological phenomena, much of it thoroughly buried since childhood, that have been causing problems or just keeping them from moving forward in their personal growth. All members of the primary group should stay alert to these insights as they come up, so that all family members can help each other nurture them and incorporate them into their personal lives while solidly supporting each other in the loving family cradle.

Inevitably, some old "stuff" of this sort will sometimes come up along with discussion of some new issue. If the new issue seems more major or urgent, of course deal with that first. But you may occasionally find that some of the old stuff underlies the new. Gain understanding of the old issues, the old traumas or deprivations or distortions from childhood, and what seemed like a serious new issue may just fade into insignificance with no effort applied specifically to that concern.

Looking at this the other way around, current issues or problems may just be superficial manifestations of deeper-lying psychological processes. A current issue may therefore seem inexplicably resistant to resolution unless underlying causes are discovered and dealt with. As with geological strata, so also in the psyche, a general working rule is that the older stuff is often more deeply buried—but the older, deeper stuff may hold insights and explanations of what is now on the surface, so excavation is worthwhile.

7.04. "Hot buttons".

What are "hot buttons"? Through the process of delving deeply into your respective childhoods, touched on in sections 6.08 and 7.03, you are likely also to discover each other's "hot buttons"—events or situations that trigger an instantaneous, unthinking, emotional response of the "fight or flight" sort, often rather ugly. These reactions originate in the limbic brain, the most primitive and the earliest evolved part of the human brain—a part of the brain very much on an instinctual, nonverbal, nonrational, animal level of functioning.

These limbic reactions are kicked into high gear in a tiny fraction of a second, before your cerebrum (where sensory input is processed and rationality and emotions reside, among other functions) can even begin to grasp what happened and contemplate what to do about it. If there is an unexpected loud bang, or something suddenly leaps into your field of vision—you automatically and instantaneously jump, and only *after* jumping does your higher brain kick in and ask, "What was *that??* What should I do about it?" It was your limbic brain that made you jump.

The limbic brain helped our species and its ancestors (and every other animal species) survive in the era of saber-toothed tigers and earlier—and its automatic response to a perceived threat can still be vitally useful to us today, but the reactions can also be quite inappropriate in modern society and in modern relationships, leading us to jump into a highly emotionally charged response to something that we later may feel was much too hasty or inappropriate a reaction. Others around us are even more likely to feel that the reaction was inappropriate.

A tragic example of inappropriate response by the limbic brain is what psychiatry has come to call post-traumatic stress disorder (PTSD), sadly common now in vast numbers of military personnel, veterans, and civilians who have been exposed to the barbarism of war. Many of these people pass us on the sidewalk or sit next to us in the bus, and their injury is not visible to us the way an amputation would be—but PTSD can interfere more than the loss of a hand or foot with the ability to get along with coworkers and deal with job situations (making it difficult to hold down a job), and to get along with family members (wreaking havoc on relationships with partners and children).

"Hot button" responses are also limbic responses, but of a milder degree than the strong overreactions that characterize PTSD. These instantaneous and seemingly inappropriate or exaggerated responses came to be called "hot buttons" colloquially because it's as if the person had a special button on their body like a button on a machine, and whenever someone pushes the button, the pre-programmed response pours forth automatically, even if it seems to make little or no sense, especially not to anyone else.

As an example, a person may have learned as a child that whenever their father said a certain phrase or assumed a certain posture, next he would fly into a rage, stirring terror in the other family members and especially the children. Or one's mother might have tended to wander off after drinking too much at home, and then one day after a drinking bout she wandered off and never returned.

Regardless of when or how they were created, "hot buttons" just lurk and wait for the wrong word or action to set off the alarms. The children of that father and that mother, after growing to adulthood, may have no conscious awareness of the emotional associations that were forged during their childhoods, unless they have been led to them through psychotherapy or another healing modality. But the child of that father, whenever they hear a close family member utter that phrase or see someone assume that posture, may mysteriously panic and become defensive or argumentative, or want to run and hide, even though the phrase and the posture have no apparent reason to lead to an outburst of anger or urge to hide. The child of that mother may now have a fear of abandonment, especially if a family member leaves home after a drink or two.

It's no surprise that these "hot button" responses can often trigger disputes with partners, because they can seem so off-the-wall, irrational, and contrary to the interests of the partnership. The problem is made worse for relationship harmony because, to anyone else, and even to the person with the "hot button", there is usually nothing visible to link current "hot button" behaviors with the events years ago that created the association. Compounding the problem further, a "hot button" response is generally out of sync with any healthy partnership dynamic; it is totally self-centered. The limbic brain has no concern whatever for anything or anybody outside itself. *"I gotta protect me! Me! Me!"*

Why is all this important in a book about personal dynamics in polyamory? If there are more partners than two (three or more primaries, or some combination of primaries and secondaries), then there are more relationships to be disturbed by the "hot button", and more individuals who might have "hot buttons"; and I have noted elsewhere that in polyamory it is more important that each relationship be on a solid foundation, as free as possible from the minor or not-so-minor irritants that a monamorous dyad can often tolerate.

How to cope with "hot buttons". Committed partners should realize from the outset that "hot buttons" tend to be very deeply ensconced in the psyche, so that it *may* sometimes be difficult to eradicate them totally; they may almost seem like immutable personality traits. (They are not.) But when a person learns of the early events that engendered their particular "hot button", that insight in itself can sometimes miraculously "switch off" the "hot button" response. If the insight does not totally inactivate the "hot button", it will at least give the person a major tool for understanding it and thereby minimizing its effect, maybe eliminating it altogether over time.

Should we get help? It is certainly worthwhile for you and your primary partner(s) on your own to try to delve into the possible underlying causes of "hot buttons". The worst that can happen from such an amateur effort is nothing—you do not get to the bottom of the "hot button", and the "hot button" continues to hold sway. But because "hot buttons" tend to be buried so deeply, usually in the subconscious so that ordinary encouragement to recall has little or no effect, professional help is commonly needed to get to the root of "hot buttons" and eliminate their effects. See section 7.14 about seeking professional psychotherapeutic or other healing help.

If you are part of a triad or larger, you and your partners together can use the "hot seat" method to lovingly probe an apparent "hot button" in one of you. (Note that the "hot seat" and the "hot button" are different concepts.) See section 9.11 about the "hot seat". If you have only one primary partner but your dyad is more psychologically aware of these processes than usual, you may also find buried treasure by lovingly and gently doing some psychological excavations on one of you. The communications techniques discussed in Chapter 6 might be helpful to you in this endeavor.

Whether you are a dyad or a larger group, be especially loving, gentle, and supportive with each other as you explore each other's psyches for "hot button" material. Be patient. Even professional psychotherapists often need a number of sessions with a client to bring these to light, using their expertise and special techniques.

7.05. *Jealousy.*

It's no surprise that jealousy is probably the single most common specific issue or problem identified by people living polyamorously, or attempting it, or considering it. The good news is that jealousy is *not* the invincible monster that it may seem to some—but at the same time it does need to be taken seriously, not just dismissed with "just get over it," or "ignore it." We just need to understand it for what it is.

Jealousy could be thought of as a specific type of "hot button" response, as discussed in section 7.04—but jealousy can manifest in a number of different ways, because the underlying past events that lead a person to feel jealousy can be very different.

Jealousy is based primarily on fear—a fear of loss of our partner to someone else. Some people with weak self-images even attach their own sense of identity to their primary partner, so that loss of that partner would be tantamount to loss of one's self—a terrifying prospect indeed.

There may be no external justification for this fear (as with other "hot buttons"); often the jealous person has constructed imaginary future scenarios based on their own internally programmed expectations (again see section 7.04). In the case mentioned in which someone attaches their sense of their own identity to their partner, obviously their identity would not really be lost if the partner leaves, only their illusory, projected identity.

Poor self-image or low self-esteem can also lead the jealous person to assume that they are likely to lose if their partner is given a choice between them and someone else. Fear of abandonment can also play a role. The jealous person may be following the "barter relationship" philosophy, whereby they (unconsciously) consider their partner to be somehow their possession or servant, someone whose role it is to satisfy their (the jealous person's) desires. They don't want to lose their "back-scratcher". See section 6.06 about the "barter relationship".

What won't work. With these pre-programmed and unrealistic expectations and fears churning away in the jealous person, expectations and fears that are buried in the unconscious, as a general rule it is completely fruitless for the jealous person's partner to try to persuade the jealous person out of their jealousy through logic or by presenting facts. "But honey, I've never given you the slightest hint that my love and my commitment for you are anything less than rock-solid. Sure, I enjoy Mary's company, but you and I have a lot more in common than she and I do, so I'd never even think of dropping you and becoming primary with her." That won't touch it.

What will work. Instead, you'll need to address your partner's old "tapes", old "programming". Find out what it was in your partner's childhood that led them to develop a low self-esteem, or a fear of abandonment, or whatever seems to be operating. This is likely to take some time, spanning several conversations.

As discussed in section 7.04, it is worthwhile for primary partners to sit down together (multiple times, if needed) and sincerely, lovingly, gently try to ferret out these deeply buried psychological influences that can lead to jealousy, but because these influences typically *are* so deeply buried, and typically unconscious, you may well discover that you need professional psychotherapeutic or spiritual healing help (section 7.14) to get to the root of whatever it is that is bubbling up and ultimately manifesting on the surface as jealousy.

If jealousy is a problem in one of your primary partners, or in yourself, be patient. An insight by the jealous person *can sometimes* lead to a very quick eradication of the feelings of jealousy (as with other "hot button" responses), but as a general rule you can expect the process of eliminating jealousy to be gradual.

7.06. If you've "cheated" in a monamorous relationship—preparations.

If you've had an "affair". Suppose you are in a traditional monamorous (sexually exclusive) marriage or committed relationship, but in spite of the promises or assumptions of sexual exclusivity between you and your spouse or partner, you have indulged in an "affair"—you've been "unfaithful"—in secret from your partner—and now you feel bad about doing this in secret. You probably consider yourself between a rock and a hard place, whether or not the "affair" is continuing. You've read section 1.01 of this book and you recognize the dangers of continuing to keep the secret from your partner. You'd like to get clean, both for the sake of your conscience and for your primary relationship. But you're afraid that revealing the facts to your partner will just bring about an emotional explosion that at worst could lead to a break-up between your partner and you, or at the least could cause considerable damage to your relationship.

There's no escaping the fact that you *have* created quite a dilemma, and you don't need this book to tell you that coming out of the situation unscathed (or not much scathed) will be delicate and difficult. It is probably little comfort to you that you are in the company of vast numbers. At this point there is certainly no guarantee that your primary relationship will come out of it undamaged, regardless of whether you choose to come clean to your primary and hope for the best, or say nothing and . . . again hope for the best.

Resolve to come clean. Ethical considerations, spiritual reality, psychology, and practicalities all clearly weigh on the side of coming clean. Beyond that, some *paths* for coming clean give you better odds than do others for emerging at the other end of your heavy discussion with an even stronger, even more loving primary relationship than you had before. What follows in this section is my own recommended approach—certainly not the only one. It should be clear that the approach described here should also work (if anything will) for other difficult situations needing discussion between the two of you.

Rehearse. I suggest that you go over all of this section plus sections 7.07, 7.08, and 7.09 on your own privately first, at least a couple of times, before broaching the subject with your partner. Also review all of the rest of this chapter for communication techniques useful in conflict situations.

Rehearse what you will say. You are not rehearsing a façade, a fiction for the stage. You are rehearsing the best way to present the *truth,* including not only the facts of your other involvement but also the truth of your deep love for your primary and your strong desire to strengthen, not weaken, your primary relationship. On the other hand, when you have the real discussion, you should sound spontaneous, not canned, so don't memorize a spiel.

Imagine how your partner might respond at various points (several possible alternatives, based on your knowledge of your partner), and rehearse how you might respond in turn.

When the time comes, you will still be nervous and ill at ease. You would be inhuman not to be. It is okay if you choke up and if you fumble over words with your partner. That will show your partner that this is really important to you, that you care for it to have a good outcome. But a little advance rehearsal might smooth things somewhat, and maybe prevent you from phrasing something in a way that you regret.

Pick a good setting. When both of you, and especially your partner, are in a good mood, tell your partner that you want to have an important discussion, so you'd like to pick a time and place together where you can have some uninterrupted time just for each other. If the two of you are already in professional counseling together, you might want to have this talk during one of your sessions. If so, the counselor would probably appreciate being alerted in advance of what you plan to bring up.

Do not choose a day that is special to either or both of you, such as a birthday, anniversary, or a holiday that is important to the two of you.

If your partner asks you, "What about?", keep your response positive but unspecific, perhaps: "There's something I'd like to tell you, and I'd like to talk with you about how we can make our loving relationship even stronger." If your partner persists in trying to draw details out of you right then, just say something like, "Well, that's why I'd like to agree with you on a good time, so we can have a good talk without interruptions or distractions." Of course, if you are at home, that good time might be right now.

Your sofa might be the ideal place, because you can sit next to each other, touching. You can put one arm around your partner's shoulder and hold hands with the other, to show tangibly that you really care. You will probably want to avoid your bed, because this kind of discussion in bed could leave bad energy fields, bad memories, contaminating all the lovely, positive energies and memories that you both associate with that bed and that room.

If you have young children, I suggest that you pick a time after they are in bed asleep so they will not interrupt you or distract you. If you have older children who stay up as late as you do, consider picking a room in your home (hopefully not your bedroom) where you can be away from them, and explain to them that Mom and Dad will be in such-and-such a room to talk about something and you would prefer to be left alone, short of an emergency. If they ask you what you'll be talking about, you can give them a truthful generality that you'll be talking about how your relationship works and how to make it better. (That will be a good example for them.)

Other options with children are to plan a time when you know they will be away at some activity, such as a school band or sports practice or scout meeting, so you know they will not come bursting in on you at an awkward moment; or you could leave your children at home (with a babysitter if they are young enough to require that) while the two of you go out to a restaurant—but of course you'll want to pick one where you can talk about private, intimate topics without being overheard. If the weather is warm, you could take a picnic lunch or supper to a local park and sit at a picnic table or a bench. Or send the children for a visit with grandparents, if that's convenient.

Having this discussion while taking a drive in your car is not a good idea, since the one of you who is driving will have their attention distracted by dealing with the road and traffic, and you cannot snuggle or make eye contact. Sitting with the car parked in a quiet place could work, but if you do this, you may want to suggest that you move to the back seat after the car is parked, so the two of you can snuggle up as you would on your sofa at home.

If you have this discussion at home, be sure your TV is off. You could play music or not, but if you do, I suggest gentle, soothing, nondistracting background music (say, classical guitar music or a harp) kept at a low volume, and it should be your own recordings, not the radio, to avoid interruptions from the announcer. If you don't have suitable recordings in your collection, I suggest that you leave the sound system off.

7.07. The actual discussion—coming clean about the past.

The "sandwich" approach to tough subjects. Psychologists, parents, and legislators have long known about a technique for getting unpleasant stuff across, whether it's unwelcome information, a foul-tasting medication, or a supplemental tax bill. Give something more palatable before and after. In our situation here, "sandwich" your unpleasant information about your "affair" between positive information, as described below.

The first "slice of bread" in the sandwich. The "sandwich" consists of first saying something nice, then the difficult subject matter, then closing with something nice again.

You can start by seating yourselves on the sofa (or wherever) so that you're both comfortable; you might want to place one arm affectionately around your partner's shoulders. You could use your other hand either to hold hands or place a hand on your partner's knee or thigh. The idea is to express your affection nonverbally.

Looking your partner lovingly in the eyes, I suggest that you first reaffirm your abiding strong love for them. Reaffirm that you've always wanted to work through any problems that come up, because the most important thing for you is to keep the two of you together as a couple, deepening and enriching your love through life. It would be good to remind your partner that you've always wanted to do that, and you still do, as much now as ever.

The middle of the sandwich—the hard part. A good way to launch into the "meat" of what you have to say is to tell your partner that you have fallen down on part of your agreement or understanding or vow to each other. You can state that of course no one is perfect, everyone slips up sometimes, but you still feel bad, you want to apologize, and you want to make things right with your partner, because you love him/her very, very much. (Throughout this discussion, you cannot say too often or too emphatically how much you love your partner!)

Then it would be good to state the basic facts of your outside relationship straightforwardly, but this basic disclosure need not take much time; avoid digressions into lateral matters. You might give your other lover's name (at least the first name, so you can easily refer to them), and how the two of you met and became attracted to each other, and the circumstances surrounding how you first shared sex with each other. If the sexual involvement has ended, or was a one-night stand, I suggest that you say when. If the involvement continues, say so.

If you do reveal your other lover's name to your partner, it would be good to ask your partner not to reveal your secondary's identity further to other people (except to psychotherapists and the like), since that is private information that does not concern anyone else.

Safe sex? It would be a good idea for you to mention whether or not you and your lover have followed safe sex practices. (If you don't volunteer this information, your primary is sure to ask.) Obviously the situation will be far better if you did scrupulously use condoms with your lover.

If you did not follow safe sex practices, I suggest that you admit it, and immediately state that you realize that this was a second transgression on your part, since you exposed your primary to the same degree of STD risk as you exposed yourself, without getting your primary's input on the matter. (This assumes that you actively share sex with your primary and do not use condoms.)

You may also want to explain why you decided that the STD risk with your other partner would be negligible (even if your current hindsight might lead you to the opposite decision). You can add that you realize now that it would be appropriate for both you and your primary to have STD testing, both now and after the medically recommended delay due to the incubation period. (See section 4.10 about the incubation period.) If you and your primary maintain separate finances, then of course you should offer to pay for the testing for both of you.

If you and your primary ultimately decide to allow this secondary relationship to continue, and if you have not been practicing safe sex with this secondary, it is still a good idea to *start* safe sex, even belatedly. Consider promising to your primary that you will be scrupulous about using condoms with your secondary from now on, unless you *and your primary* decide otherwise. See section 4.08 for further discussion.

The other "slice of bread" in the sandwich—restating love and commitment. After giving the basic facts, I suggest that you state once again that the person now sitting beside you and into whose eyes you are lovingly looking, the person you are now having this difficult talk with, is still the most important person in your life (well, maybe excepting the little darlings asleep now in the other room, or practicing the halftime formations with the rest of the high school band—and they're among the most important reasons for working through this and salvaging your relationship and making it even stronger). You want more than anything to make things right with your partner, you might want to say. You can add that you know that the best thing for the little darlings is for the two of you to stay together, if you can work things out. You can apologize again—and, oh yes, you can restate your unwavering love yet one more time. You're asking for your partner's forgiveness, and asking for help in figuring out where the two of you can go from here, what you can do, together, to make your shared life even more loving, enriching, and solid than it has been.

You are going to have to give this sort of reassurance of your love and commitment to your partner repeatedly, not just now and in the near future, but ongoing, not just in words but (even more importantly) in your actions, your behavior. This is imperative in order for you to (at least partially) rebuild your primary's trust and faith in you, which you have damaged.

Your partner's response. Your partner might respond to your revelations with anger, or surprise, or with appreciation at your frankness and your reaffirmed love and determination to work through whatever difficulties may arise; or with some combination of these and other emotions. Your partner may be relieved that you didn't have something worse to reveal, such as an intention to separate.

7.07

There is another possible way in which your partner may respond. After your revelations, he or she may give you a sheepish grin, squirm a little, clear their throat, and tell you that your confession gives them the courage to let you know that they have a similar confession of "infidelity" for you!

At first blink, this turn of events might seem like a doubly tough situation, but in fact it makes it easier for both of you. We will treat this eventuality in section 7.09. In the remainder of this section we will assume that your partner makes no such similar confession.

If your partner is angry. If anger is your partner's response, I suggest that you try diligently to retain control over your own emotions, or at least your expression of them (this time), and avoid returning anger for anger, because that can quickly spiral out of control. Venting is good, but anger reverberating between two or more people is nothing but destructive and renders any communication virtually impossible. Rather than trying to listen to and understand what the other person is saying, the angry person will be spending that time ignoring the other person or trying to come up with a hard-hitting rebuttal—the worst possible way to try to communicate and reach agreement. If *you* remain calm and cool and apologetic in your responses to your partner's angry outbursts, and if you keep reaffirming your love and your commitment to this relationship, odds are good that your partner will soon calm down as well and start to engage in constructive dialogue as you are doing.

Remember first that, whatever are the past emotional dynamics between your partner and you, your partner is fully entitled to be angry with you now. Remain calm and contrite. I suggest that you keep restating your apologies and your love and your determination to work with your partner to rebuild your relationship on healthier, more solid ground. Stay calm as you correct any misstatements of fact that your partner may make in the heat of anger—or just let the misstatements slide for now. You might make a mental note of them so you can clear up any misunderstandings later. I suggest that you ignore any insults or character slurs that your partner may make in the heat of anger.

Promise full openness and honesty from now on. At this point, you have cleared your conscience by admitting what you've done, by giving full information even if belatedly. But your partner may now be at the nadir of fear and anxiety, suffering from a shocking and unexpected blow to their trust in you and their belief in you as an honorable, trustworthy person deserving of their love and respect. Your involvement with another lover raises the specter in them that you might be thinking of leaving, that you no longer find your partner attractive—and they may harbor such feelings at least subconsciously even if you have reassured them (as hopefully you have been doing) of your continuing love and commitment.

Having gotten your confession off your chest, your next job is to start to rebuild your partner's trust in you and respect for you—absolutely essential if the two of you are to remain together in any loving way.

You can start by assuring your partner (yet again) that your love for them remains as strong as ever, or stronger, and you've now learned your lesson about withholding information from them, and you promise fervently never to do that again. ("Well," you say smilingly, "I might not blurt out in advance what present I've gotten for your next birthday, but other than that sort of thing, my heart is now a totally open book to you. You have my solemn promise on that.") I suggest that you say that you will volunteer any information that you feel is relevant to your shared relationship, and you will answer fully and honestly any questions you get, now or later.

Please note that I did *not* suggest that you hastily promise never to share sex with anyone else, but that you promise never again to *withhold*

7.07

information from your partner. The pain caused to your partner, and the damage caused to their trust in you, comes ultimately not only from the broken vow but also (even more so) from the fact that you have withheld information, maybe lied and told half-truths, in order to conceal the "affair". The question of whether the two of you will be open for outside sexual relationships is still subject to further discussion at this point, either during this talk or at another time (soon).

I also suggest that you assure your partner that you have no thoughts about leaving, but on the contrary you want very much to work together through any difficulties that may arise, so you can continue to be a loving couple together. You can cite as evidence of your strong good will the fact that you wanted to have this difficult talk with your partner, rather than just rocking along hoping that your partner would never find out, or (worse) walking out without ever explaining why.

It would be helpful for you to answer any questions from your partner fully. If you are asked if you promise never again to "cheat", "be unfaithful", or have sex with anyone else, you can say that you'd like to talk over that question very carefully together—but that whatever the two of you end up deciding *together,* you'll abide by that—unless the two of you *together* change that agreement still further in the future. You want your shared relationship to continue to come first in each other's lives.

Condoms for you and your primary? If you have not practiced safe sex with your secondary, your primary may well ask that the two of you start using condoms until you can be sure again, after the incubation period and after testing, that you are both disease-free. It would be good for you to agree to this, not only because you caused the problem in the first place, but also because it is wise from the health standpoint (because you may have picked up something and not yet passed it on to your primary). Your agreeing to condoms will also be another indicator to your primary of your good will to work together in your partner's interest and the common interest.

7.08. *Continuing the discussion—looking to the future.*

Where from here? Assuming that your partner is still talking and working with you at this point, the next step is to revisit the relationship agreement that you have between you (whether or not you have made that agreement explicit). This could be done immediately, if you both feel you still have the energy for it and if time permits, or you could set a time for another discussion, picking up where you leave off with this talk. A whole series of discussions could develop, spanning some time. This is a good thing, because it shows that you are both willing to invest ongoing work to strengthen your relationship.

You and your partner may not even realize that you have a "relationship agreement"; it may be tacit, based on "what everyone does" (that is, "forsaking all others", etc., even if you never explicitly said as much to each other). You may call it your "marriage vows", whether or not there were such words in your ceremony. It may just be what each of you tacitly *assumes* to be your shared views about how a couple "should" relate, because "everyone knows that's how committed couples relate."

See Chapter 5 about the relationship agreement. Since this issue has come up between you, and assuming that you both do have good will to rebuild things between you, now would be an excellent time for the two of you to work together to develop an *explicit* relationship agreement, preferably in writing, as discussed in that chapter—not during this first discussion, unless you both have enormous personal energy and determination, but soon. Developing and agreeing on your relationship agreement will probably take more than one discussion session, as described in Chapter 5.

7.08

If the two of you decide to defer this next phase of your discussion to a later time, I suggest that you set a definite date and time now if at all possible, in the near future—say, tomorrow evening after dinner or after the kids go to bed, or the first evening free for both of you. Write it on your family calendar or into your handheld or whatever method you use to keep track of important appointments. Of course you can change the appointed time later if circumstances require, but do not just agree to discuss it at some unspecified future time, and do not let it slide with repeated reschedulings because other things come up in life. Other things *always* come up in life. This is important. Give it priority. The two of you need to be sure to finish what you have started here.

Will our relationship be open or closed? When the two of you do consider the next step, either immediately or at a later date, the most fundamental question is whether or not the two of you will agree together to allow either of you openly and honestly to develop emotionally and sexually intimate relationships with anyone else. Of course our mainstream society immediately jumps to the answer, "Certainly not! People just don't do that!" But this unthinking reaction citing the nebulous "people" or "they" does not have to be the final word. You have your own two lives; you are grown-ups now; and you can decide this question for yourselves, after discussing the options and ramifications and (most especially) your own feelings, carefully and respectfully and lovingly.

This is essentially a yes-or-no question—to be either sexually open or not. About the only conceivable middle ground here might be to allow sexual "playing" or "petting" with others, stopping short of actual genital intercourse. Again, that's up to the two of you.

The possibilities and options for couples who wish to allow themselves outside sexual involvements are described in broad outline in section 2.03.

If the decision by the two of you is that full sexual intercourse with others *will* be allowed, then there arises a wide range of possibilities as to details, which you and your partner will need to discuss and agree on, probably not all in one sitting, and subject to revision based on experience and how you each react emotionally to real-life involvements that arise.

Close this talk with a "thank you". When this first discussion between your partner and you seems to be winding down, I suggest that you thank your partner from the bottom of your heart for their willingness to listen to you and share their own views and work with you in order to move beyond this current situation and strengthen your relationship. You could say that you look forward to further sessions about getting specific with a relationship agreement, so that future missteps hopefully can be avoided and the two of you can continue to build and strengthen your relationship for a long, long time to come.

Of course a wonderful way to cap off this discussion and reestablish a positive, loving field between the two of you would be for you to head off to bed together now and really give that mattress a good thrashing. If this isn't practical for whatever reason, you can at least snuggle up with your primary when you are in bed; just before your last good-night kiss, you can give them some nice, affectionate caresses, say once again how much you love them, and thank them again for being willing to work with you on this.

If your "affair" (secondary relationship) is still active at this point. In this case, ethics or fairness calls for you to keep your other lover (let's call them your "secondary") informed of your discussions with your spouse or primary, even though, if there is a conflict of interests, of course your primary relationship must take precedence, even to the point of terminating your secondary relationship if that's what you and your primary agree to. But one thing at a time.

7.08

In section 7.06 we hypothesized that you had decided to come clean with your primary, have the tough talk, and work with your primary to build a better foundation for your relationship. This point, when you had decided to talk with your primary but had not yet done so, could be the best time to let your secondary know of your intentions, especially if your relationship with your secondary is fairly deep and caring. If you let your secondary know in advance of your upcoming talk with your primary, then you will need to contact your secondary at least one more time (even if the outcome is to break off that relationship), in order to share with your secondary what you and your primary decided. Or, if it was decided that you may continue the secondary relationship, then of course you will want to pass that happy news on to your secondary.

The other alternative, not contacting your secondary at all until after you've had your talk with your primary, means that, if the decision with your primary is to rule out secondary relationships, then you will need to break the news that the relationship is ended in that one contact with your secondary. This might not be such difficult news for the secondary to receive if the relationship is not very deep, but could be if the relationship is substantial. If the secondary relationship is substantial and if you and your primary decide to be monamorous, letting your secondary know in advance that the heavy talk with your primary is coming up could soften the blow.

Just as with the talk with your primary, you may want to find a quiet, private place to have your conversation with your secondary. In the real world, of course, you may have to settle for a phone conversation. Email or an electronic chat should be your last choice of options for these talks, since the electronic text media totally lose the emotional content of communication expressed through tone of voice, physical gestures, etc.

You can explain to your secondary that you feel you need to disclose the facts to your primary—and that may include revealing the secondary's identity, or at least the first name—and last name too, if your primary asks (since you will agree to answer all questions). Your secondary hopefully will realize without being told that they really have no control in this situation, since they should realize that your primary relationship must take priority in your life; that's what "secondary relationship" means. Even so, common-sense empathy will call for you to be as gentle and considerate as you can in explaining the situation and your views to your secondary.

You can assure your secondary that you will ask your primary not to reveal your secondary's identity to anyone else (except a professional counselor if relevant), since that is private information that does not concern anyone else.

Whatever you do, if your secondary relationship is to be broken off, it is good for you to inform your secondary *somehow,* if at *all* possible, even if that relationship is not very substantial or deep. I feel it would not be caring just to stop phoning and electronic chatting, leaving your secondary totally in the dark about what caused you to disappear. That will leave them wondering what *they* did that so thoroughly angered you that you could not even bring yourself to make one more contact to explain your anger. Of course nothing of the sort is the case, which is why it would be very unkind and unfair to treat your secondary in this way.

Having your primary meet your secondary. Regardless of whether you and your primary decide to live polyamorously from now on, you might want to consider offering to introduce your primary and secondary to each other, if they do not already know each other. This would be more for your primary's benefit, since their feelings are the more important in your life, but certainly your secondary might also like getting to know your primary. A friendship could even ensue between the two of them—one of the delightful benefits of the polyamorous life.

The friendship would be good even if you decide not to live polyamorously. If you and your secondary do not continue to share sex, the two of you could also continue to enjoy a nonsexual friendship.

When you offer to your primary to introduce your secondary, you can point out that the unknown tends to loom larger in the imagination, especially if the unknown is thought of as negative or threatening. This is true not just in personal relationships but in all of life. Learning the facts will shrink the balloon back to real size.

Your primary may be wondering just what sort of person your secondary is, if they could lure you into bed against your explicit or assumed vows. It would be easy for your primary to imagine some extreme sex-pot (of the appropriate gender), or someone extremely scheming and unscrupulous and selfish—or all of the above, and more. Introducing primary to secondary would let your primary see that your secondary is really a fairly ordinary person—probably with ordinary looks, not porn-star material; fun to be with, of course, not the devil incarnate.

And, of course, your secondary may also be curious about your primary.

If your partner is unwilling to work with you, or unsure. After the hard part of your talk (the part between the "two slices of bread" of the "sandwich"), your primary may simply take a negative attitude about you or your shared relationship, at least as an immediate reaction, and claim not to be interested in working with you to rebuild your relationship on a better foundation. They may not know how to react immediately, feeling angry and numb.

Do not be discouraged by this. Keep your own attitude upbeat and positive. Keep saying "I love you" to your partner, and underscore this with deeds—a bouquet of flowers or a single rose, cards that say "I love you", fixing a special dinner for your partner—you get the idea. It may take a while to bring your partner back around.

Another good option at this point, if your partner seems to be having trouble with the information that you've disclosed and with continuing to work together, is to suggest that the two of you seek professional counseling (or your primary may suggest it). This topic is discussed more completely in section 7.14.

7.09. Continuing the discussion—if your partner also confesses to "infidelity".

Section 7.07 describes the situation where you arrange a heart-to-heart talk with your partner to come clean about your own prior undisclosed sexual activity (when the two of you have agreed, or it is assumed, that your relationship is to be monamorous), and that section notes that your partner might sheepishly respond with a similar confession of their own. You would be in a comparable situation if your partner initiates the confession about their own secret "affair" and you have an undisclosed "affair" of your own to reveal, as discussed in section 7.10.

Don't ignore this. Although both of you in this case have violated your mutual agreement or understanding, in fact your situation is easier to resolve now than if either one of you alone had committed that sort of indiscretion. It would be a mistake, however, for the two of you to assume that no resolution or further discussion is necessary, reasoning that you are both still in the same place with each other—that "the score is even".

It might seem that neither of you needs to forgive the other in this situation. But you both *have* gone against your relationship agreement, and so it would be better for your relationship if you *both* forgive each other. This may well be a rather light-hearted forgiving, but do it anyway. You'll both probably feel better for it afterwards. You will both *certainly* feel better now about having gotten your pair of dark secrets into the open, and the sky did *not* come crashing down!

Where from here? The next step for both of you at this point is to recognize that you have both fallen short in two ways: breaking your explicit or tacit understanding not to engage in outside sex; and not communicating with each other about it (before now). These two failures actually go together, as does the solution. People in the mainstream often "just can't bring themselves" to reveal this sort of personal failure to their partner—and if they conclude that they don't have the strength of personal character to make that confession, they *may* feel that much more temptation to indulge in such transgressions.

But you and your partner can develop a system for communicating fully with each other, embodied in a relationship agreement, which could include the privilege of outside (secondary) sexual involvements for each of you, under conditions negotiated and agreed upon by both of you. By doing so, of course the two of you are moving your relationship out of mainstream monamory (sexual exclusivity) into the realm of polyamory. When you do this, the communication will come much easier for both of you (maybe after a little practice), and any secondary relationships will be happy and guilt-free because they are done within the parameters of your relationship agreement.

7.10. If the "affair" was your partner's in a monamorous relationship.

You learn or suspect that your primary partner has had an "affair". What if you and your partner have had a sexually exclusive (monamorous) relationship, explicitly or by tacit assumption, and your partner lets you know, or you find out, that they have been sexually involved with someone else? You may come to suspect it, even if you are not sure.

7.10

Your partner may invite you into a discussion along the lines described in section 7.06. If they do not, you could suggest to them that you talk about it, in some comfortable, quiet place and at a time when you can be reasonably sure to be free of interruptions, as described in section 7.06. Do not just slough it off or say, "That's okay, honey, it doesn't bother me," and go on with life. That sort of response on your part could give your partner the erroneous impression that you don't care much about your shared relationship or about what your partner feels or does.

If your partner immediately promises never to share sex with anyone else again, you could respond something like, "Well, I appreciate that offer, but that may not be necessary. There are other options. That's part of what I'd like to talk with you about, when we have a good time and place."

Your partner's revelation. When the two of you do have your discussion of the details of this situation, right then or within a day or two, it is likely to follow a pattern similar to the one described in sections 7.07-7.08, except of course that your two positions will be reversed. Listen attentively while your partner lays out the basic facts. You can give nonverbal indications of your love and support, such as sitting on the sofa so that you touch each other, with an arm around your partner's shoulder and your other hand holding theirs or resting on their knee or thigh, and maintaining eye contact.

Your response. When your partner has finished disclosing the basic facts, I suggest that you say first that you very much appreciate their coming forward to you with this information, and reassure them that your love is still as strong as ever. You could say that your love is strengthened just by the fact that they chose to bring you into the picture, even though it was after the fact. You can add that you would like to work together to build a more solid foundation for your relationship, including finding a way to keep each other better informed of important information as you go through life together.

Moving on from here. In a way similar to that described in section 7.08, I suggest that you tell your partner that you intend always to give them complete and honest information, not withholding anything or telling half-truths that might lead the other person to false conclusions. You can ask your partner to make a similar commitment to you; you can assure them that you'd much rather have complete information than to feel that you are not always told things, maybe learning about things later, as happened this time. You can add that this even extends to information about other loving, sexual liaisons that they may want to get involved in.

Chapter 6 discusses in detail how to communicate and other relationship skills. It might be well for the two of you to go through that chapter together. There are also many other books available with guidance for couples about relating with each other in healthy ways. If the two of you do not already have an explicit relationship agreement, I suggest as the next step for you both that you develop one, as discussed in Chapter 5. See Appendix A for suggestions about books and other resources.

Safe sex? You will probably want to ask your partner if they practiced safe sex with their other lover, if your partner did not already volunteer this information. If the answer is "no", I urge you to restrain your anger if you feel it (for now).

Ask your partner if they discussed their lover's state of health, and the lover's habitual degree of caution with other lovers, before proceeding without a condom. (This discussion would be similar to the discussion about whether you and your partner agree to fluid-bondedness with a secondary partner—section 4.11—but after the fact.) If the answer satisfies you that the risk is acceptably low, then you might choose not to make a further issue of it. If the information about the lover's state of health and habits is less than satisfactory to you, or if your partner has not even discussed this with their lover, then I suggest that you state firmly that you would like for both of you to get STD testing promptly, and to be tested again after the incubation period (see section 7.07 and section 4.10).

Is it continuing? You may want to ask your partner (if not already volunteered) if their other relationship is still active, or has it ended or was it a one-night stand. If it is continuing, and if safe sex was not observed up to now, and if the two of you agree to let this relationship continue (see section 7.08), then you may want to ask your partner to insist on condom use henceforth with the other lover, unless or until *you two* decide that the other lover is safe enough that you can agree to forego condoms, according to the criteria in Chapter 4.

It is also completely appropriate, if you wish, for you to ask to use condoms with your primary until testing and the incubation period can reassure you that you are both disease-free.

Wrapping up the discussion. As in the case when the outside relationship was your own (section 7.08), when the discussion seems to be winding down, I suggest that you restate to your primary that you very much appreciate their coming forward to you with this information, and that you still love them as much as ever, if not more for deciding to bring you into the picture. You can reaffirm your commitment to keeping this relationship primary, and to working together to keeping it sound and satisfying.

Even after this discussion, your primary may have some remaining feelings of guilt or self-deprecation for handling the situation badly—for getting sexually involved with the other person in the first place, or waiting as long as they did to inform you. You can alleviate this by continuing to give your primary extra indications of your love and support over the next days and weeks—and ongoing. You could bring them flowers or a rose; give them "I love you" cards; fix them a special dinner; no doubt you can think of other extra things to do for them that you know they will like.

7.11. *Violations of a polyamorous relationship agreement.*

Let's say you are in a polyamorous relationship and you have violated some provision of your relationship agreement, or you learn or suspect that your primary has done so. The situation here is similar in some ways to the situation in which you and your partner had a monamorous relationship and one of you had an outside sexual involvement in violation of your agreement for exclusivity. The solution would then also seem similar—have a talk about it, as described in earlier sections of this chapter. To a considerable extent, this is true.

The main difference may seem like the trivial one that it was a different agreement that was violated: in the first case, the agreement not to share sex with anyone else, in the latter case, some provision of your relationship agreement—say, your agreement always to use condoms with anyone else, or to get approval from your primary partner before sharing sex with a new secondary partner.

There could be more to it in the subtleties, however. In mainstream culture, because the agreement or vow of sexual exclusivity is universally assumed for committed couples unless agreed otherwise, some people at least may take a somewhat cavalier attitude toward infractions. "Well, most people have affairs. I'm glad it's out in the open now, but we don't need to talk about it further. It's over and done with." In polyamory, in contrast, appreciable effort always goes into developing a relationship agreement between two or more primary partners, and so an infraction could be seen as calling for more serious attention.

I agree that a violation of a relationship agreement by someone in a polyamorous dyad or larger primary group should be taken seriously by the parties involved—and that's because the agreement itself is an important contract between the parties involved. At the very least, there needs to be a discussion of what provision was violated, how each primary partner feels about it, and what steps might be taken in the couple or group hopefully to avoid a recurrence. You may wish to consider whether to revise that provision in the agreement, if one or more of you feel it is too restrictive or for some other reason.

7.12. *Hidden psychological resistance.*

Sometimes in a couple or larger group, one partner (A) may suggest something (adopting polyamory, or anything else), and the other partner (B) may go along with it, though sometimes not really whole-heartedly. Their agreement in spite of lack of enthusiasm could have any of several causes. The reluctant agreement may stem from a misguided notion that this is the best way to preserve domestic tranquility. (The notion is misguided because things "shoved under the rug" in this way tend to pop out again later, causing even more unpleasantness than was initially averted.) B might sincerely agree initially, but has second thoughts later, for any of a number of reasons.

Whether B's initial reaction is complete enthusiasm or some reluctant agreement or anything between, B's later growing misgivings can put B into a feeling of being in a bind. B may feel they can't go back now on their earlier agreement. If the agreement was to try polyamory, A quite likely by now has gotten into one or more secondary relationships, and to go back on that agreement now would force A to call off the new secondary relationship(s). If B's trust in A's honesty is less than rock-solid, B may fear that A will continue the outside relationships anyway, as secret affairs.

So what is B to do in this situation? B might ask to revisit the question with A, and maybe change the agreement. Or, B could just quietly continue to go along, on the surface, but might offer some form of resistance either consciously or unconsciously. (This is what psychology calls "passive aggression".)

The resistance can take many forms, either clearly related to the issue at hand (in this case, A's secondary relationships) or totally unrelated. Since scheduling each date with a secondary calls for calendar coordination with the other primary partner, B might consciously or unconsciously come up with "schedule conflicts" as reasons why A can't be with the secondary at that particular time. If the relationship agreement between A and B calls for preapproval of a secondary partner by the other primary partner, B might find reasons not to approve various potential new secondary partners for A.

So if you are "A" in this scenario, or if you are A's secondary, and if it seems that your attempts to schedule get-togethers between A and the secondary are thwarted a great deal, passive aggressiveness *might* be behind it. Or it could simply be that A, or A and B together, really do lead such busy lives that scheduling with anyone else is difficult, and there are no unconscious roadblocks being shoved out into your path. (Poly people do seem to be the type who lead very full lives, and not just in the realm of relationships.)

7.13. Moratoriums.

Section 6.04 mentions that early in the developmental phase of a new relationship, a couple may decide to *temporarily* refrain from other relationships while they are working on developing their own. A similar kind of moratorium can be very helpful as well at any later stage in a primary relationship, when issues arise that call for the primary partners to invest substantial time and energy into their resolution.

Purpose later in a relationship. Although a moratorium early in a new relationship is generally for the purpose of allowing the new partners to focus on getting to know each other and fleshing out the details of their relationship, a moratorium in a well-established relationship can be for any purpose that calls for a large investment of the partners' time and personal energy. It can be an issue that has arisen among them. It can be some other endeavor (shared or not) that is expected to demand much time and energy for a limited time, such as moving, a death in the family, or welcoming a new baby into the home.

For a set period. A moratorium at this later stage, as with one in a new relationship, should be for a set time or until a set calendar date, not just left open-ended. When the time expires, consider whether circumstances now make it appropriate to lift the moratorium, or whether the moratorium should be extended (again for a fixed period).

Options. Another similarity to moratoriums early in a relationship is that a moratorium at this later stage can either call for a suspension of all current secondary relationships for the duration, or allow those to continue while not allowing any *new* secondary relationships to be started (because new relationships of any sort demand extra time and energy).

Suggested by a secondary. If you are in a secondary relationship with someone who has a primary partner, and you become aware of issues between the primaries, you could yourself suggest a moratorium on your secondary relationship to allow the primaries to focus more of their energies on their issue.

Another very loving thing that you as a secondary could do is to offer to talk together with the primary partners, as a third party, perhaps as a mediator, an outside listener, who genuinely cares about both of the primaries and who therefore wants to see them get over the present hurdle. You could do this with or without suspending your sexual involvement, as you all decide is best.

7.14. Professional counseling or healing help.

Choose carefully. If your issue relates to polyamory and if you decide to seek professional counseling from a psychotherapist, relationship counselor, or clergy, or healing from a spiritual healer, either on your own or with one or more partners, be careful of your choice, because at this writing many professional counselors and healers are not yet trained in dealing with issues related to polyamory, and may even view polyamory, or multiple relationships of any sort, as itself a problem, a pathology, something to "cure" you of. (Homosexuals faced the same difficulty until not many years ago, and no doubt still do, especially with unenlightened clergy.)

While adept spiritual healers can wreak healing wonders, sometimes almost instantaneously (in contrast to psychotherapists, who sometimes may require months or years to obtain partial results at best), at this writing there is no system in place for accrediting or evaluating spiritual healers; anyone can hang out a shingle. Therefore, if you wish to try for this form of healing, get a guarantee of money back if you feel you have not been helped (as some offer). A spiritual healer that I know voluntarily offers this money-back guarantee to new clients who come to her.

As the potential client, it is completely appropriate for you to ask the therapist or healer some questions about their attitudes before agreeing to come in for your first paid session. If you do go in for a session, whether with a psychotherapist or a spiritual healer, that first session is not only for the healer to learn some basics about your situation, but also for you to assess the fit between yourself (yourselves) and the healer. Of course there must be good rapport between yourselves and the healer.

If during the first session, or later, you come to feel that rapport is going to be a problem for you, it is better to let them know that fact, in person or by phone. The healer may suggest that you continue for at least one or a few more sessions, to see if better rapport can be established. This is reasonable. But if now or later you come to feel that there is not a good fit between you, let the healer know that you have decided to seek help elsewhere, and why.

Don't hang back. Don't hold off from seeking professional counseling or healing just because you might choose someone who is not poly-friendly. Most of the psychological problems, concerns, or issues that arise in poly relationships are general ones, not limited to polyamory, and any competent psychotherapist or healer would be well familiar with them in nonpoly contexts, and therefore should be able to help you with your situation, even if your particular situation does have poly content.

Even if your concern *is* one that has a unique poly twist to it (say, interactions between yourself and your primary's secondary), it is better to seek professional help if you are having difficulty resolving it on your own, because, first, a less-than-100% chance that the healer will be knowledgeable and sympathetic is still better than the zero that you will have if you don't go at all. Second, even if your chosen healer turns out to be unfamiliar with and/or unsympathetic to unique poly situations, consider that you will be doing the poly community a service by showing the healing professions that the poly community exists and their psychological problems deserve sympathetic professional attention.

Lists of poly-friendly counselors. Some local poly groups maintain a list of professional psychotherapists or other relationship counselors in their area who are recommended to the list by other polyamorists as being not only competent but also sympathetic to polyamory.

If your local poly group does not do this, you might wish to suggest that it do so—and, as always, what better way to get that accomplished than to volunteer to take care of that list yourself?

7.15. Polyamory support groups.

As a middle path between professional healing and therapy and just struggling among yourselves, some local polyamory groups sponsor self-help groups, modeled loosely after twelve-step groups such as those pioneered by Alcoholics Anonymous. Even if sympathetic professional counselors and healers are known locally, a self-help group can be very helpful for dealing with lesser problems that do not really call for paid professional help.

If your local poly group does not sponsor a self-help group, you might consider starting one. This section describes how to arrange such a group, as well as how to run a session.

Getting set up. These poly support groups meet at a regular place and time, typically once a month. The place can be a meeting room of a public library or of a sympathetic religious congregation, or other friendly or at least neutral venue. Your local public library system may have a policy of allowing free use of their meeting rooms by local nonprofit organizations—which your poly group certainly is.

If you prefer not to reveal the polyamorous nature of your group or meeting to the library (though there should be no reason not to), you can use a phrase something like "relationship support group" in talking to library personnel and where the library's form asks for the purpose of the meeting or of the sponsoring group. This is entirely honest, and it may secure you a free meeting room.

Conducting a session. Rather than being an unstructured conversation, the support group meetings have a moderator, whose job it is to see that everyone has a chance to speak who wishes to, to keep the group from digressing into matters unrelated to resolving specific poly-related personal issues that people bring to the group, and to remind the group at the beginning and end that everything said in the group should "stay within these walls"—it's confidential. This encourages people to discuss very intimate, confidential, possibly embarrassing situations in a safe and friendly atmosphere before the group.

Details of how these groups function can vary. Stick-on name tags are a good idea. Encourage (but do not require) people to put at least their first names on the tags. Typically the chairs will be arranged in a circle, since the group size should not be larger than a dozen or so, to provide an intimate atmosphere. If more than around a dozen people show up, there is obviously a need! In this case you might want to try to split the group into two, meeting at different times and/or places.

Start on time, or close to it. Late-comers may be admitted. The door of the room should be closed, for privacy, but unlocked, so late-comers can walk in without disturbing the session by requiring someone to get up and open the door. Tape a sheet of paper on the door as a sign, saying something like "ABC [acronym of name of poly organization] group—members come on in." (Members of the ABC group will not need further identification of the group on that sign. They'll know from ABC's internal publicity channels what the group is about, and that's why they came. People not members of ABC who happen to walk by and see the sign do not need to have their curiosity aroused by more detailed information on the sign and possibly decide to come in, creating an awkward situation.)

The moderator opens the meeting by introducing him/herself as the moderator and explaining the ground rules for the meeting (confidentiality, stick to the topic, mutual support and respect, everyone may speak, etc.). As an ice-breaker, the moderator may then invite everyone, going around the circle, to introduce themselves (first name or nickname is enough, so everyone can refer to each other), including a self-description in a few words—perhaps how long they have lived poly and what their current poly living situation is (or are they just poly-curious), living singly, or in a poly dyad, in a triad, etc.

7.15

After going around the circle for introductions, the moderator asks if anyone has any poly-related personal concern or problem that they would like to bring to the group for discussion. If this is any session beyond the very first, probably at least one person familiar with the process will raise their hand to speak and present an issue for the group.

If it is the very first session for this group, and maybe for later meetings as well, the moderator may need to speak for a few minutes in general about the sorts of poly-related situations that are appropriate to bring to the group, and how the group should respond. The moderator might cite something from their own personal poly experience. "For example" (the moderator might say), "suppose one of the primary partners in a poly couple is experiencing some jealousy when the other partner is out on a date with a secondary. Or suppose someone wants to schedule a date with a secondary at a particular time but that would create a scheduling conflict or somehow be awkward in the primary relationship. What sorts of suggestions would any of you here this evening offer to someone who told us they were having one of these problems?"

After people discuss these hypothetical problems for a few minutes, the moderator can again invite anyone in the group to present a real-life situation that they find themselves in. If silence reigns (the moderator may need to offer some encouraging words), the moderator can suggest another hypothetical situation, a real situation from the moderator's own life or that they've heard about (respecting privacy), or a discussion of any of the many subjects from poly dynamics, or ask if anyone else wants to suggest a topic.

The moderator needs to be alert to imbalances in how people speak. It is natural that different people have different speaking styles—some jumping in before someone else has quite finished, others hanging back so that they never get to speak before someone else takes the floor. If there is a chronic interrupter or someone who always wants to dominate the discussion by jumping in with their own response to something, or if there is someone who seems never to open their mouth (especially if their facial expressions suggest that they have something that they would like to say), the moderator needs to take action, perhaps specifically addressing that less assertive person and asking them if they have any comments they'd like to make on the subject at hand. ("George, I got the impression that you had something going through your head just now. Is there anything that you'd like to share with the group?")

The moderator can politely remind the entire group (avoid speaking directly to the offending stage-grabbers, since this should not be a personal criticism before the group) that everyone present should have an equal turn to have their say. "Because everyone will have their turn, we want to be especially sure not to interrupt anyone who is speaking. If something that someone else says prompts you to say something in response, that's great, but please raise your hand and wait till the current speaker is finished."

If the problem persists, a good solution is to use a light but easily visible object such as a stick (maybe with a ribbon tied around it), a bottle, a flashy and amusing hat, etc. You can refer to it as "the speaking stick" ("speaking hat", etc.). Only the person holding the object (or wearing the hat) may speak. When that person is done, they hold the object out before the group, inviting anyone else to take the object so they may comment.

If the group uses a "speaking stick" (anything of that sort), obviously the moderator will still have to be alert to anyone jumping in when they don't have the stick, or hogging the stick and taking more than their share of time with their turn of speaking. It is appropriate for the moderator to politely interrupt someone talking on and on and remind the group that others may also wish to speak.

A "speaking stick" (etc.) can also be useful in larger groups, even if there is no problem with imbalances in speaking styles, because with larger groups there can be the problem of several people politely raising their hand to speak at once, and then jockeying to figure out who speaks in what order. The moderator can be alert to which hand went up a fraction of a second sooner, and invite people to speak in order, using the "speaking stick", or arbitrarily choosing order by pointing to people and saying, "Okay, let's hear from you next, and then you, then you."

Closing. About five or ten minutes before the scheduled ending time of the session, the moderator should remind the group that they are approaching time to end, so any current discussions can be brought to a close. A good way to close is to go around the circle again, as at the beginning. Starting with the moderator, each person *briefly* gives their impressions of how the session went. Was it helpful? Did it help build a sense of community and empathy within the group? Is there anything that anyone would suggest doing differently about how the group was run this evening? Would people recommend this to their poly friends who were not present this evening?

After going around the circle for final comments, the moderator can suggest that everyone stand side-by-side in a circle and put their arms on the shoulders of the persons on each side, in a group hug. An alternative is to take hands for a moment while still seated. This seated connection is preferable, of course, if anyone present uses a wheelchair or crutches.

7.16. Growing out of a relationship.

When all is said and done. Let's say that you and your primary partner(s) in a dyad or larger primary group have struggled with an

7.16

issue. You've talked and talked, and you've tried all the communication techniques and issue-resolution techniques that you could find in this book or elsewhere. You've sought professional counseling. The issue remains unresolved, and one or both of you feel that, in the absence of a resolution, you'd be better off going your separate ways rather than continuing to stay together.

Of course this situation is common to all varieties of relationships, not just in polyamory. But, yet one more time, the situation can be more complex in polyamory, because there are more possible variations.

This section will look at some of the possible dynamics that apply for *poly dyads,* which can be somewhat different from the dynamics for traditional *monamorous* dyads that break up. The dynamics of breaking up for a *triad* or larger primary group are considered in section 9.12.

The two people in a poly couple preparing to break up will need to deal with the same issues as a mono couple, pertaining to dividing their shared assets, deciding which of the two will move elsewhere (or whether both will move); if there are children, deciding who will have custody and how ongoing involvement of the children with both parents will be handled; explaining the situation to friends and relatives; etc. Efforts should be made to keep both partners on as cordial a basis with each other as possible.

However, when one or both members of a poly couple have secondary partners, the new question arises as to how each secondary partner will relate with each of the former primary partners. If one or both primary partners are bi, the secondary partner may have had a sexual as well as a warmly loving relationship with both primary partners. Even if the secondary partner has shared sex with only one of the primaries, often the secondary will at least have been good friends with the other primary.

7.16

Whether the secondary has shared sex with only one or with both primaries, the parties involved in the secondary relationship are likely to want to continue that relationship—and ordinarily there will be no reason not to. If only A shared sex with the secondary, they are likely to want to continue, but the secondary and B are likely also to want to continue their nonsexual friendship. If (as often happens) all are involved in the same local poly organization, they will need to be able to continue to interrelate cordially at group functions.

Some traditional couples, upon breakup, fall into the petty, childish pattern of continuing to try to put the other former partner down among friends, relatives, or even their own children, trying to establish themselves as "right" and the former partner as "wrong", trying to establish blame. Hopefully, polyamorous people as a rule will be more mature than that (greater maturity and awareness has been necessary for conducting their poly relationship, if only for a time). The existence of secondary relationships is yet one more reason for former primary partners, now separated, to behave in a civilized, mature manner toward each other and about each other, so that the entire network of involved people can continue with their lives in a harmonious, positive energy.

A secondary relationship is ended. Because secondary relationships are typically less involved and deep than primary relationships, ending them should also usually be less involved. Normally there is no shared property or personal possessions; no children together. There are still things to consider, if either or both secondary partners decide to end that relationship, at least in its sexual aspect.

Will they remain nonsexual friends? This is usually a good option; it simply brings the relationship down to a somewhat less intense, less involved level than when the two were sexual lovers in addition to whatever emotional energies were involved.

If the separating primary partners or the secondary partner have children, sometimes the children will have met and had involvements with the other adults, if one partner visited the other in the latter's home, and may have become involved to some extent in that family's activities. If this is the case, and if these visits and activities are to be terminated, courtesy to the children requires that it be explained to them that Mom or Dad has decided not to have as close a friendship with "special friend" Alex or Barb, although they remain friends (if this is accurate). All but the youngest children will understand from their own experience that friendships can wax and wane.

At the very least, if there has been any sort of ongoing dating relationship between two secondary partners, and if one partner decides to call it off, common decency would require that person to let the other person know that they had decided to pull back from a sexual involvement, or whatever the situation is; and to give at least a little general explanation of the reasons. Don't just stop calling, unless maybe the relationship never really got off the ground to begin with, so that there is little to call off.

~ 8 ~

Day-to-Day Living

Contents:
8.01. Overview.
8.02. The tyranny of the calendar.
8.03. The closet and the outside world.
8.04. In the closet or out, and to whom.
8.05. Ways to be out of the closet.
8.06. Your children's schools.
8.07. Religious affiliation.
8.08. Children of single parents and in dyadic poly families.
8.09. Networking.
8.10. Organizing a local group.
8.11. Political activism.
8.12. Giving public presentations.
8.13. Understanding bigotry and dealing with it.

♥ ♥ ♥

8.01. Overview.

How does ordinary day-to-day life differ in a polyamorous family from life for anyone else? This chapter will look at routine poly concerns such as scheduling, interactions with the rest of society, children, and involvements with other polyamorous individuals and groups.

8.02. The tyranny of the calendar.

Love isn't limited, but time is. A common saying in the poly community is that love is infinite, but there are only 24 hours in a day,

8.02

7 days in a week. A polyamorous person's appointment calendar, or the family calendar on the wall, can get quite full, trying to fit in dates with secondaries along with all the meetings, soccer practices, doctor's appointments, birthdays and anniversaries, and whatnot that are on everyone's calendars, poly or not. In my experience, poly people tend to be active and busy, and not just with dates. When you're on the phone with a secondary trying to find a time to get together, this can be discouraging.

Some science fiction scenarios envision another dimension of time at 90° to our ordinary space-time dimensions; you can do a temporal "side trip" by stepping into a booth, pushing a button, spending an arbitrary amount of subjective time in that alternate temporal dimension; then you return and step out of the booth and the clocks in your own universe will show zero time elapsed. Those with sufficient spiritual development can visit times in the past and future as well as places distant from where their body now is, and other dimensions. But those dimension-shifting booths in fiction are—well—fiction—and most of us lack the training or innate abilities for those inner travels to other planes of time or who knows what, so for us this limitation of available time is just something we must live with and work around as best we can.

So how do we manage it? We need to be flexible, and we need to schedule well. Understanding and a sense of humor among all partners, primary and secondary, also helps.

Flexibility. Flexibility means being willing to see someone or do something at a time that might not be your first choice or the other person's first choice. Of course it's basic that the primary relationship always takes precedence, but primary partners can also be flexible in occasionally yielding a time slot when the primaries might have done something together, or just spent time together at home, if thereby one of the primaries can arrange something with a secondary that would otherwise be awkward or impossible.

However, primaries should be careful not to bend over backwards *too* far in compersively facilitating things for their primary partner and that person's secondary. If you find yourselves doing this too often, you may want to sit down with each other and look at whether one of you is being a bit submissive, not self-assertive enough. If both or all of you are too quick to yield time to allow your primary partner(s) to do things with secondaries, are you undermining the primacy of your primary relationship?

Of course it's inevitable that sometimes you will put something on the calendar (involving a primary partner or a secondary, or just yourself) and then later something else comes up that you want to do (again, with a primary or a secondary, or just yourself) during the same time slot. Flexibility also involves being willing, not grudging, to reschedule things so that you or a partner can fit something into the schedule. Rescheduling blends into "scheduling well", which we will look at next.

Scheduling well. Scheduling well, or scheduling efficiently, means arranging things in their best place on the calendar. Some things (say, a hike) can be done at any of a number of times; for other things (say, a concert), only one or two times may be possible.

Think of packing a suitcase for a weekend trip. You may start by tossing your bathroom bag into a corner of the suitcase, but then realize that you're left with an odd, L-shaped space where your shirts will not fit. So you pull out the bathroom bag, put the shirts into the only place where they will fit, and then you put the bathroom bag on top of something else, so that everything now meshes together compactly with little wasted space.

You can use a similar technique with time as you do with space. If you want to schedule something that can be done at any of a number of different times (say, a shopping errand or a doctor's appointment), think carefully before planning to do that in a block of time that might be the only time that your secondary would be able to see you—or might be a time when you and your primary want to go out to dinner, a concert, or a movie.

You can also make a positive thing out of coordinating scheduling with your primary by taking into account times that your primary wants to schedule time with their secondary in scheduling things for yourself, either things that you want to do alone or maybe with your own secondary or a friend. When your primary is away would be a good time to pull out your favorite recording of that bagpipe band or gamelan that drives your primary bonkers.

8.03. The closet and the outside world.

Relationship to mainstream society. In our imperfect human societies, in different ways in different times and places, there are certain norms that people are expected to fit, and also ways in which personal latitude is allowed. At times in Europe and in the Americas, everyone was expected to be Christian (or even one particular variety of Christian), and Jews, Pagans, those following native spiritualities, and others (or Christians not of the dominant variety) had to keep quiet about their spiritual path under threat of torture and death. At times in the United States, it was okay to be Caucasian, not okay to be of African ancestry or Oriental (though one could hardly be "in the closet" about ethnicity). Of course there are numerous other examples in different times and places.

Mainstream society in North America in recent times has had the norm that loving relationships should always be between one man and one woman, so that homosexual couples, and loving groups of more than two, have had to choose between the closet or public censure or worse.

The proscription against gays and lesbians seems to be gradually lessening (although it certainly has not vanished altogether), thanks in large measure to the conscious decision by many gays and lesbians to be "out" about their homosexuality and to confront mainstream bigotry on the matter.

The unexamined assumption that only two at a time can love may also be starting to crumble, as the polyamory community grows and becomes more visible and better known, and as many polys individually are coming out of the closet—but this societal norm against any number larger than two is still very strong, so that polys do need to decide whether, or to what extent, their poly lifestyle will be publicly visible. Sometimes public censure can be mild, as when someone chooses not to associate with a poly person; sometimes it can be much more serious. Chapter 10 examines some of the more common legal hassles that one can experience just by being visibly polyamorous, and also examines what you can do about it.

Dyads or multi-adult families. Poly dyads (in which either primary partner may also have one or more secondary partners) find it much easier to stay in the closet if they wish, since to all outward appearances they are just like any other family in the neighborhood. Even if the dyad is two men or two women, they are still the comfortable norm of two together. If either or both primary partners have secondary relationships, these are typically not visible to the rest of society.

Multi-adult families really have no option to be in the closet, at least in their residential neighborhood, their religious congregation, etc., since they will be seen together coming and going, here and there. There are, however, things that a multi-adult family can do to facilitate their acceptance in their local community and more broadly. This is discussed in section 8.05.

An exception for triads (or larger poly groups) exists to some extent for these poly groups embedded within an intentional community. The outside (mainstream) world sees simply the community, and ordinarily would have no way noticing that, say, three members of that community live and love together. The poly group might then be able to keep their existence in the closet if they wish. Of course, other members of that community itself would be well aware of the poly grouping.

8.04. In the closet or out, and to whom.

As noted in section 8.03, if you are a dyad, you have considerable latitude about whether you will be totally closeted, totally open, or somewhere between. It is also often possible to be closeted in one or more aspects of your life, open in other aspects. Your own degree of being in or out of the closet is essentially a matter of personal preference, although outside factors may influence your preference. We will look at those factors in the rest of this section and in sections 8.06 and 8.07. Note, though, that you and your primary partner(s) will have to reach agreement about whether and how to be out of the closet, because it is generally not possible for one of you to be out to a degree different from the other(s) of you.

Criteria to consider. In general, is each of you in your primary family the type who does not like to stand out in a crowd as being different in some way, or are you comfortable letting others see that you march to a different drumbeat?

Are your relatives and friends mostly of a conservative or judgmental mindset such that they would raise their eyebrows and look down on you for loving more than one at a time openly and honestly? If so, how do you feel about that? How important to each of you is it to maintain warm relations with those narrow-minded relatives and your current cluster of friends? Of course you can make new friends more in harmony with your own views and lifestyle, but you are stuck with these relatives for the rest of this incarnation!

In the workplace. Do you have a sense of whether your situation on the job might be affected by your poly lifestyle? Do you work in a place where your job tenure depends on the whim of your boss or higher up the hierarchy, or do you have some job security against dismissal for such irrelevancies?

I have always been open about being poly, including on the job, and including when I lived in a quad. (I did have job security, and I don't think my supervisors cared anyway about how we each led our personal lives.) A former primary partner of mine was generally out of the closet but chose not to reveal her poly lifestyle to her coworkers, because she was a nurse in a Catholic hospital, and not only was she concerned about possible official disapproval, but her coworkers were shocked to hear her tell them that she had actually gotten into a hot tub with several others, and no one had any clothes on! After that, my partner decided (probably prudently) not to comment to her coworkers about her various secondary relationships, trips to poly conferences and camping weekends, and the like.

8.05. Ways to be out of the closet.

Degrees of being out. You can be out of the closet in subtle ways, or in other people's faces, or anything in between.

If you don't want to be secretive (in the closet) about your polyamory, but you also don't want to be a campaigner on the front lines, you can acknowledge your polyamory in personal conversations (including email, online chats, etc.) when it happens to be relevant to conversation, in the same way that mainstream people might comment on doing something with their husband or wife, a cousin, or a friend. For example, if someone mentions a current popular movie, you might comment, "Oh yes, I saw that last Saturday night with my secondary, George," or "Oh yes, I haven't seen that yet, but my secondary George and I plan to go see it next Saturday evening."

Another very nice and popular way for three together (a triad or a dyad plus a secondary) to attest quietly but effectively to their polyamory is to be seen in public walking hand-in-hand-in-hand. Three-way and four-way group hugs in public are also nice.

Bumper stickers, T-shirts, and pin-on buttons are a somewhat more active way of being out. For example, one button declares: "I ♥ > 1". That pretty well sums it up, and you can't get more concise!

It's a cliché that there is strength in numbers. At the time that the thirteen North American colonies declared their independence from England in 1776 and started calling themselves the United States—but still faced a war with England to make their independence stick—the American revolutionary Benjamin Franklin once remarked, "We must all hang together, or assuredly we will all hang separately!"

It's just as true now. Especially in these days when a substantial segment of mainstream society actively opposes permitting any polyamorous lifestyle or anything else not from their own particular cookie cutter, under pain of incarceration and worse, it is important for polys as a community to band together, not just for the social opportunities but for protection.

See Appendix A for how to find existing global, regional, and local polyamory groups. If there is no local group near you, section 8.10 suggests ways to start one in your area. Section 8.11 discusses ways to be politically active. Chapter 10 discusses legal hassles and other legal concerns for the poly community. Section 8.13 discusses polyphobia and various forms of bigotry that we may encounter from time to time.

Give an "open house" party. If you are a newly formed or an existing multi-adult family and you are moving into a new neighborhood together, you may be concerned (maybe with good reason) about how well your new mainstream neighbors will receive you. Will they shun you, and urge their children to shun your children at school and on the playground? Worse, will they check the local zoning and lodge a complaint against you if they discover that your neighborhood is zoned for a maximum of two adults per household?

As section 8.13 notes, there is no sure-fire antidote to polyphobia any more than there is for other forms of bigotry, but becoming known in your neighborhood as good, decent people can go a long way. In other words, rather than trying to be secretive about your family structure (which is next to impossible anyway if you are a triad or larger), or presenting a hostile front, actively invite your new neighbors to get to know you. Then become active in local civic groups working for the betterment of your community one way or another.

When the quad that I lived in was fairly new and had just moved into a large home (quite comfortably large enough for four adults and five children) in an upscale neighborhood (where such large homes are typically found), we, too, were concerned with how our neighbors would receive us. In order to prevent their imaginations from going into high gear based on ignorance, we decided to take positive steps to introduce ourselves to our neighbors. By means of flyers that we left on people's front doors for a couple of blocks around, we invited our neighbors to an "open house" at our new home on a Sunday afternoon, saying that we were new in the neighborhood and would like to get acquainted with you, our new neighbors. We put all four of our names at the bottom.

We dressed in our formal finest for the occasion—the women in nice dresses, my co-husband and myself wearing suits and ties.

We had a pretty good turn-out—which *might* have been due in part to the fact that people in the neighborhood were probably curious to see the inside of our *house,* which was a very grand-looking mansion with three floors (not counting the full basement) dating from about 1860, give or take a decade or so. All the other houses in the neighborhood were modern. But even those who may have come mainly to see the house also got to meet the four of us and our five children, which was *our* purpose.

We did not say anything that would explicitly identify ourselves as a quad—nor did we say anything to mislead them. We did *not* introduce ourselves by saying things like, "These are my wives Angela and Barbara, and this is my co-husband Carl" (names changed). We simply gave our first names and left it at that: "Hi and welcome! I'm Pete, and this is Angela, and Barbara, and Carl. And the kids here are...."

Of course we offered everyone a tour of the house.

We can never know to what extent that open house may have helped, but we never had any problems with the neighbors. (None of them became ongoing friends either, but at least we got no hassles from any of them.)

8.06. *Your children's schools.*

Do you have school-age or pre-school children? What face will you present to your children's schools? Keep in mind that even if you circumspectly list only one mother and one father for official interactions with the school, and even if you've cautioned your children that some people might not understand or approve of the kind of family life we have here at home, children do tend to talk (well, so do we adults), so that news that you are a multi-adult family (if that's the case) will probably get out at your children's school.

When I lived in our quad, the oldest two of our combined five children were of school age. We decided to be totally up front with the school when we bought a house together, moved into it, and enrolled the kids in their new school. We listed all four adults with the school office as serving in the parental role, so that any of the four of us could sign permission slips, report cards, and the like, and the school could discuss personal matters about either of the children with any of the four adults. The school accepted this without blinking an eye, and just wanted to be sure they got all four names down correctly in their records. (This does not guarantee that your children's school will be equally accepting!)

8.07. *Religious affiliation.*

Are you members of a religions congregation? How well does your denomination accept families that do not follow our mainstream society's norm of one man and one woman? If your denomination officially opposes forms of the family other than that norm, you will need to decide for yourselves whether you are comfortable, as a poly couple or multi-adult family, letting your poly lifestyle be known in your religious community when your clergy and your fellow parishioners might condemn you and be openly hostile toward you. Will you want to enroll your children in the religious education classes, knowing that your children (as at school) will be likely to reveal your poly lifestyle one way or another even if you are trying to stay in the closet?

If your denomination or your congregation is one of the ones that welcome lifestyles and lovestyles other than that norm of one man and one woman, you are fortunate. If there is dissonance for you here, even if you resonate well with this denomination's approach to spirituality, of course you must decide which will take priority, your comfort with the spiritual path or your discomfort with official opposition to your lifestyle.

You may want to reexamine just how much you really resonate with a path of "spirituality" that would condemn you or others just for your choice of who you love, or how many. Knowing that some organized religious denominations do accept diversity of this and other sorts, you may want to look around to see if you would feel more at home (and would feel more comfortable enrolling your children in the religious education classes) in a different denomination, a different religious community. Another alternative, of course, is to remain unaffiliated, pursuing your spiritual development (for yourself and your children) on your own, with the help of friends, spiritual groups, workshops, books, etc.

8.08. *Children of single parents and in dyadic poly families.*

See section 9.06 about children in multi-adult families. See section 8.06 regarding interactions with your children's schools (whether your family is a dyad or larger). This section has to do with what you tell your children and how you interact with them if you are a polyamorous dyad, that is, you are a couple and one or both of you have secondary relationships, or if you are a single parent.

The single parent. Your situation is relatively simple, because, if your children have reached a certain level of maturity, they will easily understand your desire to date as a means to finding a new mate, as well as for your current social enjoyment. However, if you date more than one person at a time (which could categorize you as a "polyamorous single"—see section 2.02), and if your children are old enough to wonder why you are not limiting yourself to one "candidate" at a time, you may need to give your children at least some explanation of your poly relationship philosophy—the older the children (into adolescence or early adulthood), the more complete your explanation and discussion. Of course this is especially important if you have a secondary relationship with a married or committed person, and your children know this.

The couple. For a couple, more questions arise. Children at some point come to learn the mainstream norm that, once a couple has been established, there should be no branching out into further romantic or sexual involvements. But even if you try to remain generally in the closet towards the world outside your home, it will be difficult to hide your poly involvements from your children, when they reach the necessary level of maturity.

When one or both of you are out on a date, what do you tell your children left at home with your primary partner or the babysitter? Do you concoct a "white lie", or do you tell them the truth about your relationship with these other persons, your secondaries?

What do you tell the children when a secondary phones your home, and one of your children answers the phone (as they like to do after they reach a certain age), and then (after you've hung up from that conversation) your child asks who that was?

I favor letting the children know what they are capable of understanding depending on maturity level, for several reasons. For one, in addition to learning that their parents are polyamorous, the children will learn that polyamory is natural and right, not something to hide or be ashamed of. For another, children are naturally very perceptive; if they are not actively told of your polyamorous lifestyle, they will probably figure it out, maybe at an age earlier than you would have guessed, and then they will wonder why you are trying to hide it from them. They are likely to assume that it is something that you are ashamed of, and again they will wonder why.

8.08

Assuming that you do inform your children that you are polyamorous, when they are mature enough to understand, they should also be mature enough to understand that not all segments of society understand or accept that lifestyle. They are likely to hear comments now and then, from their friends, from the mass media, or elsewhere, that reinforces the mainstream notion that polyamory is wrong.

Therefore, at the same time that you inform your children that you are polyamorous and why, I suggest that you also discuss with them how you prefer to relate with society at large. If you have chosen to remain in the closet, you can explain that fact to your children and your reasons for that choice. If you are out of the closet, you can tell your children that they may occasionally hear comments criticizing their parents' lifestyle. You can suggest ways in which they can respond to such comments. When they have reached this level of maturity, you can suggest that they use the same general approaches as are suggested in sections 8.03 and 8.04 for poly adults.

"Special friends". For young children who do not yet understand romance and sex, you might want to refer to your secondaries or your primary's secondaries as "special friends". ("Mom is on the phone right now with her special friend Dave." "Dad is out this evening with his special friend Ella.")

Of course, kids of a certain maturity will pick up on the term and ask, "Why is this friend *special?*" If they come to you with such a question, that may be a sign that they are mature enough for a basic explanation of love, romance, and sex—and a more complete explanation of polyamory, including the sexual aspects and the ethical aspects of openness and honesty. Or you could just fall back on the honest but more limited response that "Your dad and I call Jim a 'special' friend because Jim and I care a lot about each other, even more than most friends do."

If you don't relish the prospect of this kind of conversation with your child, of course an alternative is to refer to your secondaries simply as "friends", not adding the qualifier "special". Even so, don't be surprised when your child asks why you spend so much more time on the phone and in person with this particular "friend" compared to other friends!

I've seen billboards urging parents to have sex education talks with their children, "because if you don't talk with them, someone else will!" The same applies to polyamory. Would you prefer your children to get their first impressions of polyamory from someone else, who may or may not be favorable to the notion, or from you?

8.09. Networking.

Local poly groups. Your life will be greatly enriched, socially and otherwise, if you can connect in person not just with one or a few with whom to develop primary and secondary romantic relationships, but also with a number of others who share your orientation or preference for polyamory. Even in casual conversation, it is refreshing to be able to toss off a remark about what you did last Friday with a secondary, or to allude to your two primaries, without getting raised eyebrows or a puzzled look in response, so that you have to fall back on explaining polyamory from square one yet one more time.

Local polyamory groups can provide that sort of ordinary social interaction with others who also understand and resonate with polyamory. These groups can provide other sorts of support and social interaction as well, such as group massage; group picnics or bike rides; and special-interest subgroups such as for bi polys, poly women or men, young adult polys or senior polys, or those in poly/mono relationships; support groups for personal issue resolution; and more.

Local poly groups also often have a web site and provide an email discussion group in which anyone can participate by abiding by basic rules of courtesy. If you are not familiar with these email groups, when you are signed up with one you can post a note to the group by addressing it to the group's email address. Your note is then received by everyone else in the group. Your inbox will bring you the commentary from everyone else. You can respond to someone else's note simply by clicking on "Reply" in the usual manner, then drafting your own comment and sending it. Your reply will to go to everyone in the group, not just the person who wrote the note that you are responding to.

Many cities and towns have established poly groups. See Appendix A for information about how to locate existing umbrella or local groups. If there is no local group conveniently close to you, see section 8.10 about forming a new group in your area.

Sometimes several local poly groups will get together to sponsor some activity. For example, there is an annual camping weekend for polyamorous people in several areas of North America that are organized by individuals from a number of local poly groups around the region; these camping weekends also draw participants from all around the broader region.

Global and electronic groups. There are also several polyamory organizations and online sites that aim to serve anyone anywhere. They provide services such as online and paper magazines, poly-focused personal ads, chatrooms, information about local poly groups, and poly conferences, among other things.

8.10. *Organizing a local group.*

Let's say you have searched for a local poly group in your area, and found nothing close enough for you to travel to. You have also looked at the global and electronic poly organization websites, and done your own online search; nothing.

All is not lost. It is easier than you might think to start your own local group.

Jump-starting a new group. There is no minimum size for getting things started. If you have one or more primary and secondary partners, or just a poly friend or two, you already have a workable nucleus. For that matter, there's nothing wrong with a "group" of one, for the purpose of getting started. Whether or not you have partners or friends that you can enlist for the effort, there are almost certainly other polyamorous people in your general vicinity; it's just that you haven't found each other yet.

Place an ad on a poly-focused personal ad site, mentioning that you're looking for other poly people in your general area to get a local group started. You may find an online ad site that offers chatrooms by geographical area. (Chatrooms and other online sites tend to come and go, so it's not practical to offer specific references in a work of this sort.) These are another way to get the word out. You can also place flyers, announcements, etc., on physical or online bulletin boards or in other venues where more thoughtful and independent-minded people are likely to see them, such as health food stores, book stores, coffee houses, college gathering places, public libraries, and the like.

Name. Decide on a name for your group. That's up to those present, of course (or even you alone, if you're starting as a "group of one"), but I suggest that the name identify (a) your city or geographical area and (b) the fact that it has to do with polyamory. The name can then end with some synonym for "organization", such as "network", "society", etc. I personally like the name "network", since it suggests the interconnections among those in the group.

For example, when I was one of half a dozen people co-founding a poly group in the area of central Maryland and Washington, DC, we named it the Chesapeake Polyamory Network (because we hoped that

8.10

the group would serve a broad area around the upper Chesapeake Bay, where no other poly groups existed at the time). CPN took off, but it tended to draw people just around the metro Washington, DC, area, with not many from Baltimore. Later, helping to get a group going in Baltimore, we named it the Baltimore Maryland Polyamory Network. (We had to include "Maryland" in the name because the acronym "BPN" had already been taken online by another organization.)

Expanding. Once you have your group identity, you can announce your existence in the same venues where you searched in vain previously for a group local to you. If you are in the U.S. or Canada, be sure to let Loving More know of your existence, since they maintain a page of links to local groups throughout the country. Look around for other poly websites that provide links to local groups. Don't overlook nonpoly sites in your area who might be sympathetic to providing a link to your group.

For an online link, obviously you need to establish a website to which the link can point. For other sorts of listings, all you need to provide is the name of your group and a personal name and email address for people to use in contacting you. Including a phone number is optional, but if you do that, you may get calls at inconvenient times. Of course you can turn the phone ringer off and let incoming calls to go voicemail, but then you need to remember to respond to your voicemail messages *promptly,* so they don't get stale.

Activities. Initially, the most obvious activity is simply to get together for talk, both informal, unfocused chat and also focused discussion of how to move your organization ahead and grow. A pleasant way to meet is in a restaurant or coffee shop. Seek out a good place on your own. The restaurant should have decent food but not be too expensive. It should be reasonably quiet, to facilitate conversation among you. It should have either a side alcove or a way to push tables together so that a group of up to a dozen or more can sit together. To check on the latter, it is helpful to speak to the manager. Restaurant managers are naturally eager to accommodate groups such as this, since it's good for their business.

Choose a regular time to meet—say, the third Wednesday of each month.

When you start meeting in this way and a few others start coming, you can talk about other possible activities that the group could do. Ask around the table what recreations people enjoy—bicycling, hiking, picnicking, boating, whatever.

A fun activity for indoors (ideally in someone's home with a big enough living room or rec room) is group massages. People divide into groups of four, so three massage one. Time the sessions (half an hour each is good), so that people can get up and stretch and wash hands, then repeat three more times so that everyone gets a turn to receive. You may decide to allow some sexual stimulation (if a given recipient wishes), but it is good not to allow the massage sessions themselves to evolve into unrestricted sex, because then it will be impossible to stop a session after half an hour and give the others a chance to receive. If some people want a sex party and you as organizer are willing, they can stay after the time scheduled for the group massage.

A book discussion group is another possibility. Ask for suggestions about a book to read (with a poly theme or not); then choose one book. Announce a time and place to get together and discuss it, allowing enough time for people to read it beforehand.

Another good activity for a local poly group to sponsor is a "support group", in which people can bring problems or issues related to poly life for discussion and resolution by the others present, in a confidential and supportive atmosphere. Support groups are discussed in more detail in section 7.15.

Holiday parties, or parties for no occasion, can also be fun.

When the group grows large enough, you can also consider forming special-interest subgroups, for example a group for those who are both bisexual and poly; one for poly women; one for men; younger or older polys; etc.

If there are one or more poly groups in other cities in your general region (say, one or two or three hours away by car), you might consider suggesting occasional joint activities with those groups, such as a conference or a weekend camping trip.

There is one potentially discouraging phenomenon that you are likely to run into, so be aware of it. It seems to be endemic in human nature, or at least very common. Most people don't want to take the responsibility even for figuring out a place, date, and time to announce a gathering, even when they have expressed an interest in gathering. They want someone else to arrange everything. Unfortunately, this tendency seems to extend to poly people as well. The following exchange actually happened in my local poly group.

Person A posted to the group's email list: "Are we meeting this month?"

I responded: "Deborah and I would be glad to attend a gathering. So, [name of A], where and when will it take place? :-)"

A replied: "AAAAAAAAAAAAA! Rash. Allergic to responsibility!"

I give A credit for being honest in self-assessment!

So be prepared to do the arranging yourself, or together with one or a few others of the more proactive members of your group, if you want anything to happen.

8.11. *Political activism.*

At this writing there has been no appreciable grass-roots social cause or movement to secure freedoms and privileges for those who wish openly to love more than one at a time, because to date there has been little public oppression of polyamorists (some, but not much). That lack of public oppression is probably due simply to the fact that, at this writing, the polyamory community as a whole simply has not been very visible. The word "polyamory" is only now coming into the general vocabulary, among people who are not themselves polyamorous.

But that situation may well change. As we in the polyamory community become more numerous, more out of the closet, and hence more visible, those of a reactionary bent, those who want everyone to be stamped from the same cookie cutter (their own cookie cutter, always), can be counted on to start inventing open ways to repress us and persecute and prosecute us.

Section 8.13 speaks of this phenomenon more from the standpoint of psychology, discussing how to relate to bigoted people one or a few at a time. Mass actions can also be taken. A successful struggle usually is based on both these prongs—actions in the political arena, and person-to-person conversations based on awareness of the psychological processes that underlie bigotry.

Within political channels. This involves communicating your interest in rights for polyamory to the elected and appointed officials in your government at all levels. It involves asking candidates for elective office what their position is on these questions, and communicating your own concerns and views. When necessary, it also involves challenging discriminatory, unfair laws or officials in court.

Another approach, of course, if you are so inclined, is to run for elective office yourself—and, if you win the election, use your position to work for repeal or amendment of bad, discriminatory laws and enactment of new good ones.

The extent to which this general political approach may see positive results will depend, of course, on the extent to which the government

8.11

of your country, province, or locality is responsive democratically and judicially to the will of the people and dedicated to preserving the rights and privileges of all component groups. You have to assess for yourself whether efforts along these lines are worth the time and energies that you would expend, or whether you'd just be spinning your wheels fruitlessly so that you would be better off using other techniques as described below.

Public demonstrations and other mass efforts. Whether or not your government is committed to rights for individuals and minorities, and especially if it is not, mass actions can be effective under certain circumstances. These can include mass public demonstrations, boycotts, and efforts to get correct information out to the general public through alternative channels when the mass media are devoted to hiding and distorting the truth. Even if news of the demonstrations, boycotts, etc., is squelched or minimized in the mass media, you can be sure that those in power will keep *themselves* well informed about these mass actions in accurate detail, if only to keep their backsides covered and preserve their power.

Personal and underground channels. These types of effort involve person-to-person communication of various sorts, by personal contact, in local groups, by means of email and other Internet channels, and (if electronic media are too much subject to official eavesdropping) by paper mail and other means more difficult to track. Electronic channels have proven to be very effective simply for getting the word out when official channels and the mass media (in lockstep with officialdom) are trying to hide the truth and present only one orthodox and fictitious version of what is happening in society.

There are two main reasons for this great effectiveness. First, as the cliché has it, no amount of darkness can suppress even a small amount of light. Second, information that is spread on the personal level expands exponentially. If one person tells (say) five others, and each of those five tells five others, etc., the numbers become enormous very quickly: One person tells five others, so now six people know. At the second round, those five tell a total of 25 more (5 × 5). Adding that to the six who knew earlier means that now a total of 31 people know. At the third round, it's 125 more (25 × 5), for a total of 156; then the total is 781; then 3,906. After only ten rounds of this process, a total of 12,207,031 people will have gotten the word. And so on. (Yes, for the purists among you, the arithmetic here assumes a simplified ideal—that no one passes the word on to someone who has already been informed by someone else. Even allowing for occasional duplication, you can see that information can spread extremely fast just by personal word of mouth.)

The Internet has greatly expanded this power of the personal word, especially via email discussion groups, blogs, and the like. It's far easier for one person to get the word out to far more than five individuals when that first person can simply post a note to an email group, which typically will have dozens or hundreds of members, not just five or so. With the same idealized conditions as above, and if each person passes information on to 100 others through an email group or a blog or something similar, it would take only *five* rounds to spread the news to *the entire human population of Earth,* and then some.

So if you live under a regime where the mass media control what you are told and not told, take heart. Your simple word of mouth is more powerful than all their forces of darkness and ignorance.

How to get the ball rolling. Many people get inspired to get involved in some social cause or movement either when it starts to impact them personally or when circumstances in general become bad enough (for example, environmental degradation). But if you personally have no experience with this sort of activity, and if you want to start a mass movement where none yet exists, how can you learn how to do it and get other people involved?

Chances are that you also have sympathies for some other social concern that has already attracted many people to its cause—environmentalism, women's rights, homosexual rights, reproductive rights, any of a number of other progressive social causes.

You do not need to be part of an oppressed group to join their cause. I became active in the movement for black civil rights in the southeastern United States when I was in my teens and 20s, even though I am white. Later I became active in the women's rights movement, even though I am male. Both blacks and women, respectively, welcomed me into their ranks for the common cause. You can fight fascism in a country from inside that country as well as from outside. And so on.

The *methods* for conducting a mass campaign of this sort are essentially the same regardless of the specific cause. Thus, you can join one group working for another cause that you believe in, and learn those methods or tactics from the leaders in that movement. Then you can apply your expertise to the movement for polyamorous rights and privileges, or whatever else comes to inspire you.

There *is* one organization now existing that stands out as working specifically for the rights of "sexual minorities", including relationship minorities such as the polyamory community. That is the National Coalition for Sexual Freedom. See section A.03.

8.12. Giving public presentations.

Certainly a good way to get the poly message across to the rest of society and to dispel ignorance and polyphobia is to look for opportunities to speak before religious services and other groups, offer workshops on polyamory at nonpoly conferences that have a theme relating somehow to personal growth or interpersonal relationships, and the like.

8.12

If you do find an opportunity to speak before a group, and if you have more than one loving partner—say, if you are part of a triad, or you are in a poly couple and you can invite a secondary partner to join you—you will get even more impact by having three of you at the podium instead of just one—taking turns speaking, perhaps. Having "reinforcements" with you will also help if you are prone to butterflies in the stomach when you speak before a group.

Of course not everyone feels comfortable appearing before a group or has good public speaking skills. But even if you have no experience doing this, don't underestimate your abilities. It is not difficult. Rehearse your talk, and get someone close to you to listen to your rehearsal and critique the contents and your speaking style, voice strength and quality, etc. (A threesome can critique for each other.) There are also professional coaches for public speaking.

If you have a small audio recorder (or can borrow one), record a rehearsal and then listen to the playback. You might be mortified to hear what you sound like to others if this is new to you, but think of this as a tool to help you hone your speaking style. If your speaking voice comes across raspy or whiny or barely audible or drill-sergeant-ish or not self-confident, these are things that you can change with intent and practice and feedback. You will end up sounding better not only when speaking before a group but on the phone or chatting in person as well.

Unconscious "fillers" in your speaking. One thing to look out for (and listening to a recording of yourself is a good way to do this) is, you know, frequent repetition of, you know, meaningless "filler" words and phrases, which, you know, some people just seem to, you know, stick into their talking so much that, you know, you suspect that they don't even, you know, realize how often they say it. You know?

Another common habit to watch for in your speaking is the extraneous vocal question mark. You've probably noticed? How some people give a word a rising inflection? Several times in the middle of a sentence? Even though the sentence is not a question? Maybe you do this yourself?

Do you use the word "like" in place of "said"? "He's like I don't know if I like want to go, so I'm like, well, I think you'll enjoy it, and then he's like, well, if you think so."

So if you make a recording of yourself speaking, when you play it back listen carefully for "you know", "like", "um", "uh", etc., as well as vocal question marks. If you find that you do have a habit of inserting lots of those "fillers" and inappropriate rising inflections into your talking, then be alert for them whenever you talk so you can stop yourself from saying them. It *is* a habit, so it will take conscious effort and practice to change the habit.

Another way to catch yourself saying these "fillers" or other bad speaking habits is to ask your partner just to hold up an index finger whenever you say your habitual filler or vocal question mark in ordinary conversation.

If using a microphone makes you nervous, then include a "prop" mike in your rehearsal—maybe a banana or a lollipop propped up in front of you, or held in your hand, which you pretend is a mike. If you have access to a real PA system, practice with it, so you get an idea how close to hold the mike in front of your mouth.

If you will be standing before the group for the real talk, then stand when you rehearse.

8.13. *Understanding bigotry and dealing with it.*

What underlies bigotry. Bigotry can be a complicated psychological process, but basically it rests on fear (one of the fundamental human

8.13

emotions), which in turn rests on untrue negative assumptions or beliefs (which the bigoted individual either imagines or, more often, picks up from others), resting in turn on ignorance, since ignorance is the fertile ground that is necessary for any sort of false view to take root and thrive. Bigotry also requires a gullible frame of mind, since the bigoted person must be willing to take as true things that other people say with little or no evidence for it.

Another common trait among bigots is either-or thinking, dividing the world up into two mutually exclusive categories, rather than seeing things on a spectrum or with gray areas. If you are not one of the good people (our group), then you are evil. If you are not blessed by God (by being part of our own religious affiliation), you are damned to hell. If you are not a patriot (agreeing with us politically), you are a traitor. And so on.

People typically learn these ways of thinking early in childhood, from their parents and even (unfortunately) from their religious training, which often indoctrinates the child into accepting ("believing") what's presented to them completely uncritically, just because some authority says so. The "authority" is always some lesser personage such as the local clergy or the child's religious education instructor, never the person revered as the founder of the religion (Jesus, Mohammed, etc.), since those founders always taught universal love, tolerance, and acceptance of people who are somehow different.

The fact that fear is at the top of that domino chain is why bigotry against specific groups is sometimes given the name "-phobia" (which is the Greek word for "fear"); for example, "xenophobia", "homophobia", or "polyphobia".

The psychological process of bigotry works the same regardless of the object of the bigotry. Thus, if you understand how someone can be bigoted against, say, blacks or women or homosexuals, you will also understand bigotry against polyamorous people.

Psychological projection. A phenomenon well known to psychology is called "projection". When a person has feelings, mild or strong, that the person considers wrong or inappropriate or uncomfortable (real or imagined shortcomings in oneself, for example), the person will often unconsciously "project" the feelings off onto someone else, either someone close such as a spouse or partner, or people in general "out there". The projecting person will not even recognize that those feelings are present in themselves, and so they'll be unaware that they are projecting.

For example, if someone is indoctrinated to believe that a married person should not feel sexual attraction for anyone else, and if that person feels some forbidden stirrings of arousal for someone other than their own spouse, quite commonly they will not recognize even that they have those feelings—but they will become jealous of their spouse even with no provocation, suspicious that it is their *spouse* who may be feeling sexual arousal for someone else. If someone is indoctrinated to believe that homosexual arousal is wrong or sinful, and if that person feels some faint (or stronger) stirrings of arousal for someone of their own gender, they may not acknowledge that they have such feelings, but odds are good that you will find that person in the front ranks of zealous gay-bashers.

Sexual arousal for the opposite gender, when one is married and presumed not to have such feelings any more, can also lead not only to jealousy but to polyphobia, in the same way as feelings for one's own gender can lead to homophobia. Both the homosexual and the poly person not only embody that which is forbidden, but these people, the gays and the polys, even have the audacity not to show any shame or remorse!

8.13

This is how the bigot thinks.

Negative stereotypes about polyamorists. Just as untrue negative stereotypes have arisen in different times and places about other marginalized groups (blacks, Jews, women, homosexuals, the tribe in the neighboring village, and on and on), there are already glimmerings of certain negative stereotypes aimed at polyamorists. We need to know what these are, so that we can give ourselves the opportunity to come up with appropriate responses when we hear or suspect any sentiments of this sort.

Some people in the mainstream appear to see polyamory as more threatening than homosexuality. The reason mentioned above—forbidden sexual desires projected onto someone else—is one reason. Another reason is that polyamorists can be seen (by some mainstream people) as personally threatening in a way that a gay or lesbian would not be. If, say, Frank and George Gaycouple come to a mainstream meeting or religious service and introduce themselves to Harold and Irene Mainstream, Harold and Irene might feel a little uncomfortable from not being sure how to interact with Frank and George, but they would have no reason to feel *personal* threat, because they know that Frank and George, being gay, would not be expected to be sexually interested in a hetero man nor in the woman.

But if John and Katy Polycouple introduce themselves—and it is publicly known that they are poly—then not only might Harold and Irene Mainstream feel uncomfortable in the same way as when they meet the gay couple, but they might feel in addition (maybe unconsciously) that a poly person might try to promote a sexual relationship with their own partner—since (so they might believe) poly people want lots of sexual relationships and have no respect for the traditional assumption that once paired off, a person is off-limits to sexual approaches. Thus either half of the Mainstream couple could feel that their own marriage or committed relationship is threatened by the presence of the poly person or couple.

If reason played any part in this, then of course we would expect this kind of stereotyping to be applied even more strongly toward swingers, who usually acknowledge that their primary interest is sex with many partners as recreation. The fact that we have not seen this phenomenon directed toward swingers may be because relatively few swingers are out of the closet about their swinging predilections.

So how do we respond to that stereotype? Sadly, as we all know, the bigoted person generally has a closed mind to any information that would contradict their preconceived notions ("My mind's made up—don't confuse me with the facts"), but the truth is still our best tool. If we suspect that we're witnessing an instance of the stereotype described above, for example, we can look for an opportunity to make clear, first, that polyamorists are not single-mindedly and indiscriminately looking for more and more sex; second, that ethics, including respect for other people's wishes, is fundamental to polyamory, so that if we meet someone in a couple that has an agreement for sexual exclusivity, that person really is off-limits for any sort of sexual approach. Not only that, but because sexual exclusivity is the most common relationship dynamic in our culture, we would *assume* that anyone in a committed relationship is sexually exclusive unless we learn otherwise.

Countering bigotry. There is no easy antidote for bigotry of any flavor, because the root causes (projection, early indoctrination into beliefs which one is forbidden to examine, closed-mindedness, etc.) all go back at least to early childhood, and all depend on unconscious processes of the mind. Thus, it is absolutely futile to resort to logical persuasion to combat bigotry. It is also futile to suggest to the homophobe that they might harbor some feelings of arousal by their own gender, or to the polyphobe that they might still feel some sexual arousal for anyone other than their legal spouse or their committed partner.

Because bigotry rests on conditioning, about the only antidote is counter-conditioning, which of course is a slow and incomplete process. The homophobe may find their anti-homosexual feelings moderated if they repeatedly see gays and lesbians who are both out of the closet and who are visibly decent, ordinary folks, caring and loving and behaving as good citizens. The same is true when a polyphobe repeatedly sees three people walking hand-in-hand-in-hand or hugging, or hears casual comments from friends or acquaintances about things the friend did with their secondary, and the like, *and* the polyphobe (again) can see that the poly person is a decent, caring person, with well-behaved children, showing their ethical values in their public activities.

We have an example of this in recent history. Through the 1960s in the United States, sex between two unmarried people was frowned upon, and for two unmarried people of opposite gender to live together was shocking. It was kept hush-hush when it was occasionally done—a tightly locked closet indeed. Starting in the 1970s, more or less, as more and more people openly acknowledged that they did these things, mainstream attitudes changed, so that sex between two singles, and cohabitation, came to be part of the mainstream norm. Yes, there is still a segment of the population that claims that everyone should remain virginal until their wedding night, but they are now such a small minority that their views seem quaint. Society does change its attitudes.

~ 9 ~

Multi-Adult Families

Contents:
9.01. Overview.
9.02. How relating in triads and larger groups differs from dyadic.
9.03. Triads.
9.04. Quads.
9.05. From pentads to intentional communities.
9.06. Parental identity and functions.
9.07. Living arrangements.
9.08. Finances.
9.09. Personal space.
9.10. Family meetings.
9.11. The "hot seat".
9.12. Leaving a triad or larger group.

♥ ♥ ♥

A triad was making its first visit to a psychotherapist's office. When all were comfortably seated, the therapist said, "So, what brings the three of you in to see me today?"

"Well," said Adam, "my two primaries here, Beth and Charlie, and I really don't have any serious problems; we all get along fine and we have a good relationship. But—well—we've been together as a committed triad for a number of years now, and somehow the excitement that we felt in the early days just isn't there much anymore. Life is kind o' humdrum for us these days. We'd like to see if we can get some of those good NRE-type feelings back again."

9

"I agree, that's certainly worth the effort," said the therapist. "Tell me, just to get things started here, what is your sex life like?"

"Oh, it's okay," Beth said. "These two guys are both hetero, so it's Adam and me, or Charlie and me, or all three of us, me in the middle. On Sunday evenings, Adam and I share sex. On Monday, it's Charlie and me. Tuesday, we have a threesome. Then on Wednesday it's Adam's turn again, and we repeat the cycle through Thursday and Friday. Saturday evenings we leave available for dates with secondaries."

"Hmmm," said the therapist. "I wonder if maybe you've all become too much settled into a routine. I'd like to suggest that all three of you try to be less rigid, more spontaneous in your life. If any of you gets to feeling a sexual urge, give in to it! Never mind what day of the week it is or whose turn it is. Try that, and come back to see me in a week."

A week later the triad was back in the therapist's office, big grins on all their faces.

"Well," said the therapist, "You certainly all look happy! How did your week go? Did you try my suggestion?"

"Oh, we certainly did!" said Charlie. "And it was wonderful! Just a couple of evenings ago, we were just starting to eat dinner, and I got this rush of loving feelings for Beth, and I was really feeling very lucky to have two such wonderful mates! I looked over at Beth and caught her eye and took her hand in mine, and then Beth reached out her other hand to take Adam's, and Adam took mine, so we were linked hand-in-hand-in-hand. And—uhh—well—I guess our combined passions sort o' took control of us all. We all stood up and together we just lifted all the dishes off the table onto the floor, and then we pulled all our clothes off and we climbed onto the table and got into some really hot three-way sex right there on the tablecloth!"

"Wow!" said the therapist. "Was it exciting?"

"Oh yes!" said Beth. "It was fabulous, having these two guys both giving me pleasure in just the ways that they know better than anyone else—and I was giving back to both of them too! But—there's just one problem."

"Yeah? What's that?" asked the therapist.

"They'll never let us back into *that* restaurant again!"

♥ ♥ ♥

9.01. *Overview.*

What this chapter covers. Chapter 6 focuses on communications and other relationship skills that are common to both dyads and larger groups. Chapter 7 focuses on conflict resolution in all varieties of polyamorous living, including in dyads. This chapter focuses specifically on dynamical features that are particular to triads and larger primary groups, including techniques for conflict resolution in groups larger than two.

Conflict resolution in a multi-adult family (three or more) can be a challenge, because of the extra complexity—but the complexity is offset by additional techniques available when there are more than two loving partners.

This chapter also discusses some other dynamics that are either special to multi-adult families or may need special attention, such as parental functions, finances, and sharing space.

Catalyst for personal growth. There is another decided benefit to the dynamics that are special to a triad or larger polyamorous family—not just the dynamics of conflict resolution, but all of the multifaceted loving give-and-take, back-and-forth-and-sideways. These processes strongly lead the individual to do lots of introspection and reassessment of their own habitual ways of thinking and feeling, which leads in turn to strong and rapid personal growth. I experienced this in my quad, and I heard my primary partners in the quad make similar observations about themselves. I have heard of this phenomenon as well from others who have experienced multi-adult family life.

So, if you are in a triad or larger primary group, and you find the interactions among you and your primary partners sometimes somewhat daunting, take heart. There are tools available to you and your partners, and you are all likely to come out the other end of your deliberations as more aware, more capable, more developed souls than you started out. In short, whatever effort you and your partners put into it will be well worth it in what you all get out of it.

Pace yourself. That said, beware of burnout. The human mind and body can only take so much pressure, work, stress, etc. There are "circuit breakers" in both our minds and our bodies to pop us out of whatever we're subjecting ourselves to in excess. Like electrical circuit breakers, they often pick times to pop that seem extremely inconvenient. If it's an electrical circuit breaker, it may decide it's overloaded when we have a lot of unsaved work on the computer, or a dozen house guests are arriving for a special dinner. The body can throw an illness or a heart attack when we're *right in the middle* of that big project that we're really anxious to get finished. (Yes, I'm taking my own advice here and not pushing myself overmuch to finish writing this book!) The mind can go into a depression or pick fights that can destroy a relationship, no matter how highly we value that relationship consciously—because something in the *unconscious* is torpedoing the relationship for its own reasons.

Certainly burnout is a factor in dyad relationships as well (poly or mono), but the added complexities that are inevitably part of life in a triad, quad, etc., make pacing oneself especially important whenever there are three or more primary partners.

Fortunately for you in triads and larger, it may also be *easier* to pace yourself than it is in many other common life situations, such as when you are one of two heads of household with children to raise, or (even more so) a single parent. You can take off for a weekend by yourself, or with one of your primaries, or with a secondary, and leave one or more of your primaries to do parent duty in your absence. You'll come back refreshed and ready to return the favor for them.

9.02. *How relating in triads and larger groups differs from dyadic.*

Emotional complexity goes up exponentially. Chapter 6 stressed that thorough communication is imperative both in polyamorous dyads and in primary groups larger than two. However, there are differences in the interpersonal dynamics within a primary group of more than two compared to a dyad.

It's basically a matter of greater complexity, resulting partly from the number of relationships involved within the primary group (completely leaving aside secondary involvements for the moment). Section 1.01 notes that when we consider the number of twosome, threesome, etc., combinations in a multi-adult family, the complexity of relationships in that family goes up *exponentially* as members are added one at a time:

2 people	1 relationship
3 people	4 relationships
4 people	11 relationships
5 people	26 relationships
Etc.	

Different quality as well as quantity of interpersonal involvement. As the sheer *number* of interpersonal relationships increases exponentially with the number of primary partners involved, there are also *new qualitative* phenomena that are possible only with three or more primaries. Actually, this fact should come as no surprise, because there are also phenomena that occur in a committed dyad that are impossible for people living alone, no matter how much they date. A committed dyad involves the give-and-take of juggling two personalities, two sets of preferences, and two individual moods of the moment, which, as everyone who has lived as a couple knows, often are not in sync, no matter how compatible the two people are overall.

Section 9.03 looks at phenomena that first arise in a triad, that is, when there are *at least* three primary partners. Section 9.04 then looks at quads in the same way, and section 9.05 considers pentads and larger primary groups.

9.03. Triads.

We would expect that in a triad the juggling of individual preferences and moods etc. will be like that in a dyad relationship, only more so, since there are half again as many people—and this is true. But beyond that, as noted above, new things start happening when there are three. This is because there is no longer an even balance of two personalities with their two sets of interests, see-sawing back and forth.

By adding one more person to a dyad, the concept of *majority and minority* arises for the first time. This is relevant not just in organizations and political entities that decide things by voting or hierarchy, but also in the interplay of personal wills and personalities in multi-adult poly families.

The existence of majority and minority does not mean that one person is going to be shoved into a corner, their desires rolled over by the rest of the family. That *can* happen, but it would be pathological if it did, and it doesn't have to. All primary partners can work together to build consensus. (Convert the see-saw into one of those playground gadgets consisting of a large spring-mounted disk with handles for several children to hold onto while they gleefully bounce the thing around.)

One positive way in which majority/minority can work in a triad (or larger) is the phenomenon and technique called the "hot seat", described in section 9.11.

Who gets the middle. One other phenomenon in triads is the obvious one of needing to decide your arrangements in bed. This is entirely up to your personal preferences—all three in a king-size bed, or two together with the third in a separate bed, or each having their own "home" bed, moving around for sex. (A queen-sized bed is fine for threesome sex, but can be a bit cramped for sleeping.)

If it's all three in one bed (both for sex and for sleeping), and if you are a sexual "V", then you will probably want the person who is the point of the "V" in the middle. If you share sex in all three twosome combinations (a sexual triangle or delta), you may want to rotate who gets the middle.

(See section 2.12 for a description of the "V" and other alphabetic combinations of lovers.)

If you prefer sex in twosome combinations (always or sometimes), then you will need some method of deciding which two of you are paired on a given night. This could be strict rotation by the calendar (as with the triad in the psychotherapist's office at the beginning of this chapter), or it could be flexible based on personal preferences each evening, perhaps based on which one of you first expresses a desire for that evening.

The latter is how we did it in my quad. You might be concerned that leaving the choice to someone's expressed preference each evening risks strife if there's disagreement. In my quad we never experienced that problem. We left it to one of us to invite a bed partner for that night. If it occasionally happened that another of us had the opposite preference (we were two men and two women, all hetero, so there were two possible male-female combinations), that person was not disappointed, because, after all, we could look forward to the company of that other partner the following evening, and we also loved the one that we were "left with by default" and so we were happy to spend this night with that person.

Regardless of sexual preferences or orientations, the odd number in a triad means that typically there are two partners of one gender and one of the other, unless of course the triad consists of three women or three men. This inequality of gender numbers may occasionally bring up gender-related questions, though I am not aware of any substantial issues in this regard.

If you are now single or part of a couple, both of you being hetero, and you're thinking of adding a third hetero partner, you may wonder whether an MFM or FMF triad works better. Obviously this is really just a matter of preference, but there is one factor here from biology that you may want to consider. A woman typically is able to have repeated orgasms and continue with sex until she is physically tired, while a man typically needs to "recharge" for a while before he can resume functioning sexually (except with fingers and tongue, of course—and except when he has suppressed ejaculation in order to achieve multiple male orgasms). For this reason a woman is easily able to sexually satisfy two men, whereas one man may find it a challenge to satisfy two women. By this criterion, and all else being equal, an MFM triad might work sexually better than an FMF triad—again, if all parties are hetero.

More time needed for family discussions. Because of the added complexities of family dynamics in a triad or larger group compared with a dyad, as well as new phenomena such as the "hot seat" (section 9.11), a triad or larger group is likely to find that they need more time per week or month (compared to a dyad) for all partners to sit down together and discuss questions about how their relationship is working, as a whole or concerning the relationship that involves a subgroup of less than all of you (one of the three twosomes in a triad, or the six twosomes and four threesomes in a quad).

This has the disadvantage of filling more time for all with what may seem like "just maintenance work", but it has the offsetting advantage of helping all family members grow psychologically and spiritually, by means of the "hot seat" or just from the exercise of thinking about these things explicitly and discussing them together.

In addition to more structured family discussions, of course you will also have plenty of informal sharing of experiences, thoughts, and feelings between and among you as you interact each day.

You're a team. As a triad or larger, you'll find that you'll be able to figure out ways to work together to take care of all of the *real* "maintenance work" of the family, thus lightening the load per person compared to what a single person or member of a dyad must do. This includes childcare, paying the bills, cleaning the house, doing the laundry and the dishes, mowing the lawn, tending the garden, home repairs, etc.

Children. Teamwork can certainly help greatly with childcare if you have children in the home—and it's likely that the children will really love having more than one or two parents around to interact with and to help them get their diapers changed, help with homework, have heart-to-heart talks about their dating relationships—as well as doing fun family things like going for a walk or a bike ride or a picnic with one or some of the parents even when other parents are busy. Don't be surprised to see your children really blossom with the extra positive adult love and interaction available to them.

Another benefit for children in a multi-adult family is that by observation they learn about diversity and thinking and living independently.

9.04. Quads.

If there are two men and two women in a quad, the potential gender balance concern with triads is absent. Again with two of each gender, and all being hetero, there is a balance of two couples for sex, in two possible combinations—in addition to threesome and foursome sexual combinations. In an all-hetero quad with two of each gender, most likely the partners will tend to pair off at least much of the time in one of the two possible MF combinations—in addition to fun in threesomes (if one partner is tired or absent—or likes to watch or wield a camera) and in group gropes of all four together.

Most dynamics in a quad resemble those in a triad, in terms of needing to meet to communicate and discuss, sharing childcare and chores, etc. (See section 9.03.)

The "hot seat" phenomenon described in section 9.11 is even more pronounced in a quad compared to a triad, since now there can be three people "ganging up" (lovingly and supportively) on one partner at a time. Offsetting this is the fact that a quad again has an even number of partners, so that (unlike a triad) there could be a "tie" of two on each side of an issue, similar to "you have your opinion and I have mine" in a dyad.

9.05. From pentads to intentional communities.

When a primary group grows to five (a pentad) or larger, another new phenomenon, or class of phenomena, starts to appear, and becomes more pronounced the larger the group grows. The group starts to show the dynamics of an organization or a community as well as that of a family. That is, one or more partners may show tendencies to move more into a leadership or managerial status, while one or more others may tend to hang back and be more passive. Parents and children will tend to identify with each other more on the pattern of the "nuclear" family, less so with all adults being co-equal "parents" to all children (see section 9.06). Subgroups and special interest groups may appear. Secondary partners, friends, and visitors come and go to varying extents, associating more with one or more family members and less with others, taking part to varying degrees in family activities, joining in family meals, staying overnight, etc. New partners may be accepted into the family somewhat more casually than would be case with a dyad or triad, and others may exit, again with relatively less effort to resolve issues that may impel them to leave.

Thus, as the numbers increase, the dynamics of the *family* tend to assume relatively lesser importance as the group tends to function more like an *intentional community* (IC). This is not necessarily a problem, depending on what family members want; but you should be aware of this if you are increasing your numbers into this range, or thinking about doing so.

See section 2.07 for further discussion about intentional communities. See section A.04 in Appendix A for contact information about the intentional community umbrella organization, the Fellowship for Intentional Community.

9.06. Parental identity and functions.

When there are children in a newly formed triad or larger multi-adult family, the adult partners need to decide whether all adults or just the "original" parents will act in the role of parent toward each child. For ease of language, in this section (only) I'll use the term "original parents" to refer to the adult(s) who were in the day-to-day or custodial parent role for a child—whether biological, adoptive, foster, or step-parent—prior to formation of the expanded family.

In a way this question is no different from that facing a single parent who remarries or forms a new committed dyad. The single parent must

9.06

also decide to what extent the new partner will identify and function as parent along with the child's original parent. As usual, however, the question can be more involved when a triad or larger committed group is formed.

There are advantages and disadvantages to doing it each way. The decision on this question may, however, be determined mostly by the age of the child when the multi-adult family is formed, or whether the child is born into the multi-adult family. A young child of course has no concept of biological parentage, but identifies "Mommy" and "Daddy" as the adults who are there and take care of them and love them. At this stage, the child can easily adjust to identify a new adult entering the household as another mommy or daddy. As the child grows and matures, of course they come to have a more fixed idea of who their "real" mom and dad are, distinguished from all the other adults that they come in contact with.

All adults as equal parents. Thus, if a child is still very young when a multi-adult family is formed, or if a child is born into a multi-adult family, it is more natural for all adults to identify and interact with the child as a parent to an equal degree, so that the child will come to think of and name each adult as a "mommy" or "daddy".

When necessary to avoid ambiguity, the child can be taught the given names at least of the "parents" of the same gender, so that the child can refer, for example, to "Dad Abe" or "Dad Bill"—though in direct address, naturally either the name or the designation could be omitted. So for example, when talking to a mother not in the presence of either father, the child might say, "Dad Bill took us for a walk in the park this afternoon." Alternatively, especially in direct address, the child could be taught to say, "Dad, may I have another cookie?" or "Bill, may I…?"

The quad of which I was a member when my children were young had a variation on this nomenclature problem that may be unusual but surely is not unique. We were two men and two women—and the other man was also named Pete! Thus it didn't help for the children to refer to my co-husband and me as "Daddy Pete" and "Daddy Pete". Our solution was to use our initials, when context was not enough to distinguish us: I was "PB", and my co-husband was "PX" (last initial changed).

Distinguishing parents and nonparents. If a child is into pre-adolescence or adolescence when a multi-adult family is formed, the child of course will already have well-formed ideas of who Mom and Dad are, and probably will not adapt readily to thinking of a new adult in the home as another parent, or will not do so completely. Of course the transition from early childhood when the child does easily identify another adult as another "mommy" or "daddy" to the stage of having a clear idea who is and is not a parent is a gradual one. If you are now forming a multi-adult family, you probably have a good idea about where your children are in this process.

If you and your partners decide not to try to establish a parental identity for new adult(s) joining the family, because your children are beyond that stage, probably the best sort of relationship between children and the new adults is simply that of buddy or good friend. The children can address the new partners by their given names, while continuing to address their accustomed (original) parents as "Mom" and "Dad" (if that is the custom).

If the new adult partners assume this sort of buddy relationship, they can still function in a parental role to the extent desired, for example, helping with homework, giving birthday and holiday gifts, acting as mentor and confidant, tending a child when sick, going on outings together, etc.

The new partners can also discipline a child from the "buddy" role, but only after carefully discussing discipline policies with the original parents so as to prevent mixed messages or allowing the child to play one adult off another. The children also need to be told by the original parent(s) that they, the parents, are extending the discipline function to the "buddies".

Both the original parent(s) and the "buddy" adults should sit down with the child or children early on, as the combined family is being formed or will soon be, to clarify to the children what role in discipline and otherwise the new adults will have. This would naturally fit as part of a family meeting including the children in which the children are informed about the plans to add one or more adults to the family, or merge with another family. If not done then, it should be done soon thereafter.

Advantages and disadvantages. An obvious advantage of having all adults in the family functioning equally in the parent role is clarity and lack of confusion both for the adults and for the children—and so the children won't get the idea that they can get away with things around one or more of the adults in the family and not around others. A possible disadvantage of this arrangement is that if the multi-adult family later breaks up, the emotional trauma to the child of losing one of several parents can be greater than if it is "a good friend" who leaves—though there will be trauma for the children in the latter case as well, which the adults should recognize. (See section 9.12.)

Identifying biological parents. When a child is born to a man and woman who live together (no other men in the household), it's natural to assume, absent information to the contrary, that the man in that home is the child's biological father. Legally, a child is *presumed* to be the child of the mother's legal husband at the time of conception (for example, for pension or inheritance rights), regardless of her behavior when the child was conceived and regardless of obvious indicators to the contrary such as different physical characteristics between the

9.06

child and the woman's husband, unless special procedures such as DNA testing are undertaken to challenge the presumed parentage and establish different parentage for legal purposes.

Since the advent of DNA testing, some studies of biological parentage have been done, and the results have shown surprisingly high percentages of cases in which a child is born to an established couple but the husband (or cohabiting male partner) of the child's mother is not the child's biological father.

When a child is born into a polyamorous multi-adult family with two or more male primary partners, the family may not care which man is the biological father; both or all men may be considered equal "daddies", as discussed earlier in this section. (Of course the child could also be the biological child of a secondary partner of the child's mother. A lesbian couple might decide to conceive a child by means of biological intercourse with a man of their choosing rather than through artificial insemination.)

There may, however, be times when it will be helpful or important to know the child's biological parentage. For example, if a possible biological parent or grandparent develops a heritable disease, it may be important to get certain medical testing or treatment for the child, or at least to be aware of the possibility that the child may also carry the potential for that disease.

There are also legal reasons (in our legal system that recognizes only one father and one mother) to establish who is *legally* the father. These reasons can include giving permission for medical procedures and other legal consents, hospital visitation rights, interactions with the child's school, child support, custody rights, and pension and inheritance rights. (Those are examples; that is not meant to be an exhaustive list.) See section 10.06 for a discussion of legal considerations regarding parents and children.

9.07. Living arrangements.

As two singles develop a closer loving relationship, at some point they typically start to think about whether they would like to live together. The same is true as a loving relationship develops among three or more adults—but (same refrain yet one more time) the situation is more involved with triads and larger groups.

If an established couple and a third person are considering whether to live together, typically the couple will consider the question between themselves, in addition to discussing it with the third person. The consideration is not between three separate people. The same is true when two couples consider forming a quad.

The options are really broader than "either live together or live separately". In addition to those choices, the members of a triad or larger group could maintain nominally separate residences but spend a lot of time with each other, including overnight. If a sexual "V" is involved, the "point of the 'V'" could alternate between the homes and beds of the two other partners.

Alternation between homes can be based on whim of the moment, or according to some schedule. I know of one primary couple with a very close (almost co-primary) secondary male partner. The primary male partner travels extensively, and the secondary male partner stays with the female partner much of the time that the first male partner is away.

Even if a group maintains two separate households, the homes can be physically very close—in the same neighborhood, or even next-door. The extreme of this variation is to buy or build both halves of a duplex home and install a new door in the partition between the two nominally separate homes. If two doors are installed in the same opening, back-to-back, then each door can be locked from its respective side, if desired, so that no one can come through the door unless parties on both sides desire it.

A similar arrangement is sometimes used when an elderly parent who needs some assistance with daily living needs to live close to adult children who can give that regular help with meals, transportation, etc. When an addition is built onto an existing self-standing house for this purpose, it is often called a "mother-in-law apartment". Something like a "mother-in-law apartment" might work well for adding a third partner to an existing couple relationship. The extent of merging of the households can vary from two completely self-sufficient living units (with kitchen, bathroom, laundry facilities, etc., in each) to just an additional bedroom and maybe bathroom, with all other rooms and home facilities shared.

Which of these arrangements would work best for your group? Obviously that's a matter of personal preference. If you do consider some variety of living together, remember that completely sharing the same home, especially when more than two people are involved, brings in more complicating factors that don't surface when people date without living together. (See section 1.05 and Appendix C.) Is each of you habitually an early or late riser and sleeper? How warm and cool do you each like the home environment? Are you clutterers or neatniks? What are your various tastes in music that you might want to play at home, or TV programs, etc.? These and similar questions can turn a wonderful dating relationship into a disaster when the people involved try to share the same home. One of the partially shared arrangements described above can be a good solution if you do run into differences of these sorts.

9.08. Finances.

The group will need to decide how they will handle finances: Will all income be thrown into one "pot", with all expenditures (housing, food, utilities, etc.), whether for the family or for one individual, coming out of that shared fund? Will there be separate "pots", one for the family and one for each adult member?

This is a matter of personal preference. It is basically no different than the question for dyads, who must also decide whether the two partners will pool all resources or have separate accounts. The only difference is again one of degree, since there are more individuals in a triad or larger group.

If the decision is for separate accounts, then there will be a separate checking account for the joint fund and one for each individual. One charge account can be designated for joint expenditures, and each individual partner can have another charge account for their personal expenditures. Each partner will need to keep two separate supplies of cash, one of joint cash and one of personal cash. (Fortunately, most wallets have two separate compartments for bills.)

For cash, you do not need to carry this down to the smallest coin, requiring two coin purses. The practice that my primary partner and I follow is to keep separate supplies of paper money, joint and personal, and merge coins. If for a particular expenditure we lay out coins, or we offer bills and receive coins in change, we round to the nearest dollar. (We're in the U.S., where the smallest paper money is $1.00. In your case if elsewhere, you can round to the amount of your country's smallest paper bill.) Coins are considered personal, so, for example, if we get back change of 50 to 99 cents in a joint purchase, we move a dollar bill from the "personal" pocket of the wallet to "joint". If we occasionally neglect to do this rounding of coins, the effect on family finances is insignificant.

My own personal preference, based on experience, is to have separate accounts, one joint account for the family and one for each adult. The advantage of this arrangement is that clearly shared expenses, such as housing (mortgage or rent), groceries, utilities, and other categories, can easily be paid out of the joint account without each primary partner having to chip in their share for each expenditure—which could lead to astronomical bookkeeping. This arrangement also avoids disputes about expenditures that individuals may make for themselves. If there are separate joint and individual accounts, then if one member wants to buy a new gadget or book just for their own amusement, or have a date with a secondary, that clearly comes out of that person's private account, and it doesn't affect any other family member, so there is no need for a discussion as to whether to make the expenditure, whether cash outlays were extravagant, etc.

If there are separate accounts, three more questions must be decided:

(1) How will each partner's contribution to the joint fund be calculated? Will each of the partners be expected to contribute an equal cash amount each month, or will it be proportional to each partner's personal monthly income (exactly or approximately), or some other formula?

If all partners are gainfully employed and earn a similar amount each month, an equal contribution from each might be simplest. If different partners earn substantially different amounts, a weighted contribution from each may be necessary or preferred. If one or more members work gainfully full-time and one or more either are full-time childcare givers at home or are part-time gainfully employed and part-time childcare givers, you may want to consider whether you want to factor in credit to the care givers for their nonmonetary contributions to the family welfare.

(2) Which expenditures are joint expenditures, and which are personal or individual? There is room for flexibility and personal preference here, so be sure to discuss this among you.

9.08

Some examples that you will *probably* want to put on the joint side are: housing (rent or mortgage and property taxes), utilities, groceries and home maintenance supplies, furniture, any outside activities or travel shared by all partners (such as restaurant meals or travel together), books and recordings that the entire family will enjoy. You will *probably* want to put these on the personal side: clothing; expenditures for personal hobbies, recreation, or travel not shared by all; dates or travel with others outside the family; and income taxes.

The gray area in the middle includes car or other travel costs, including mass transit for commuting to work. These costs include car payments, fuel, repairs and maintenance, and insurance.

If your group considers that cars are owned individually (which is especially likely if someone joins or forms a family and already owns a car), then it is reasonable to consider that car payments as well as secondary car expenses, such as fuel, insurance, etc., are all chargeable to the individual owner. If cars are considered as a shared family property, then you may decide to charge all those expenditures to the joint account.

(3) Sometimes one or two partners, fewer than all of them, want to buy something for the family. If the money amount involved is substantial, all partners should agree before the expenditure is made. On the other hand, it can be awkward to call a family meeting before every minor expenditure of joint funds. Therefore it's a good idea for all partners to agree, as part of their financial arrangement, on a maximum single cash expenditure from joint funds that any partner can make at one time without having to consult the other partners.

At this writing, my partner Deborah and I have agreed on fifty dollars (U.S.) as the maximum that either of us may spend of joint cash at one time without first consulting the other.

All these details about family finances, after they've been agreed on by all partners, should be put into the relationship agreement (see Chapter 5).

9.09. *Personal space.*

This is another piece of the dynamics that is also shared by dyads, but becomes more prominent in multi-adult families.

You all rejoice in being a family together—but everyone also wants some alone time now and then, some space (literally or figuratively) that they can crawl into, where they can be alone and do their own separate thing. Different people want different amounts of alone time and space, and they want it in different ways.

As more people are added to the family structure, it becomes steadily more important to give this matter *conscious* attention, and maybe come to a group agreement on times when each partner may be absent. Otherwise, partners will just quietly disappear now and then for a while, and that could be at times when their presence in the group is really wanted for some task or for something fun.

One or more partners might come to feel that another partner is "disappearing" too often and for too long, or conversely that they are "in my face" too much. One or more partners may come to feel that family demands are pressing in on them too much, depriving them of the "space" that they want. A conscious agreement can head off this sort of issue.

It is also important to establish private and shared *physical space.* If a partner has their own bedroom, that room naturally becomes their private "space". If a bedroom is shared with one or more other partners, something else will have to be arranged. If, say, two partners share a bedroom, the agreement for private physical space could be a "time-share" sort of thing. That is, it might be agreed that one of those two partners has the right to be alone in the bedroom at certain times, the other partner at other times.

If a partner has a special hobby or interest that involves a separate space, this is another way to provide for this personal need. One partner may like to putter in a home workshop in the basement, or play a musical instrument, or paint, or work a potter's wheel. You may decide to set aside a special place as a music or art or pottery studio.

But these personal activities do not necessarily have to involve separate physical spaces designated for the purpose. I enjoy playing the dulcimer, and my primary partner is an artist. I have my dulcimer set up in one corner of the living room, and she has her easel in another. If we're both in the mood to do our personal things at the same time, she can listen to me practicing the dulcimer, while I can look over and see the progress on her canvas.

9.10. Family meetings.

The quad that I was in spent quite a lot of time (it seemed to us at the time) sitting in "family meetings" in our living room after the kids were in bed, discussing how things seemed to be working among the four of us. Occasionally these sessions involved conflict resolution, although a large majority of the time was spent simply trying to sort out the unfamiliar psychological and spiritual dynamics that we were experiencing as a multi-adult family, since we had no guidance or path markers whatever, and we knew of no one else doing anything of the sort.

We had no schedule for these meetings; we just sat down together for a talk whenever we needed to try to sort something out, which seemed remarkably often, even though things mostly went well for us.

We didn't at all mind the time used in this way. It was another form of relating together and strengthening our bonds.

For yourselves, you might also decide to have a talk just when you feel the need; or you might decide to schedule a regular time for a "family meeting", maybe once a week. Having a regular meeting time would not necessarily involve the kind of unhealthy rigidity which the therapist at the beginning of this chapter talked about; a certain amount of structure can be good, as long as you aren't rigid about it. An advantage of regular meetings of this sort would be to *proactively seek out* any issues among you while they are small, rather than waiting till one of you comes to feel strongly enough about something to call a family meeting to resolve it. If you have a regular meeting time, and you all sit down at the set time and discover that you have no concerns to put on the agenda, then you can spend a few minutes looking for some way to celebrate together how well things are going for you!

If you have children in the home who are mature enough, it would also be a good idea to have "family meetings" that include the children, to give them an opportunity to share their observations and their concerns and questions—and to give them a good role model for their own future adult lives. These family meetings with the children would be separate from and in addition to the adults-only family meetings.

9.11. *The "hot seat".*

I have experienced this myself, in the quad in which I lived for a time. As already noted, if it had been just my one primary and myself and we failed to reach agreement after good-faith discussion, I could easily say, "You have your opinion and I have mine, and it appears that we'll just have to agree to disagree." But if I were in a triad and *both* of my primary mates lovingly said, in effect, "Pete, you really need to look at this in yourself," I could not reasonably fall back on asserting that my view has equal weight with the combined views of both of my mates. If I'm in a quad and *all three* approach me in that way, the effect is that much stronger.

In our quad we sometimes referred to this as the "hot seat phenomenon", when three members of the quad lovingly and compassionately confronted the remaining member on some issue or personal "growing edge". All four of us in that quad experienced being "in the hot seat" at one time or another. As a consequence, all four of us experienced rapid and substantial psychological and spiritual growth. Speaking for myself, I am very glad to have had that experience and that growth.

Holding a "hot seat" session does not have to be a conscious decision—and in our quad, it never was. My mates did not say, "Okay, let's put Pete in the 'hot seat', because he just isn't seeing this in himself." Rather, we'd be having one of our family meetings for looking at the dynamics occurring among us, trying to sort things out, and it would just happen to come out that one of us was a minority of one on some question, or one of us was manifesting something psychological that impacted the rest of us.

In this kind of discussion, certainly finding a majority and minority view on some question is not the end of the discussion. A family is not a parliament that votes and the majority rules. The person in the position of minority of one may have a valuable insight that the others just haven't seen yet, and a little friendly discussion can bring the others around to that way of seeing things. It could also be a matter of valid differences of personality among the partners.

Where the "hot seat" does show its unique value is if one of the partners has some personal "hot button" or weakness or blind spot or denial, an area where some personal change and growth really is appropriate, for that person's benefit and for the sake of smooth waters for the whole family. Examples (among others) might be if someone is chronically late, or messy, or controlling, or careless about leaving lights on when they leave a room. If a person with a bad habit such as one of these is in a dyad, the one other partner may have a hard time persuading the first partner to mend their ways (to "grow" is a better way to put it), since they are evenly matched in number. The chronically messy or late person could counter-charge that the other partner is too much of a neatnik or a clock-watcher. But two or three partners can bring that many times as much weight to bear when they lovingly press their partner to make the effort to be punctual, not to strew dirty dishes and clothing in the living room, to be more egalitarian, or whatever.

9.12. *Leaving a triad or larger group.*

The following discussion is most apt in the case of dissolution of a triad or quad. For groups larger than four, section 2.05 and section 9.05 note that the larger the group, the more the dynamics of the group begins to resemble that of a community instead of a domestic partnership. It becomes actually easier and simpler in larger groups (say, half a dozen on up) for one or a few people to leave, as it can also sometimes be easier to join.

If one partner in a triad (A) decides to leave, a dyadic relationship between B and C still remains, or could remain. This means that A owes it to B and C to discuss the transition thoroughly, to enable B and C to decide between themselves if they wish to continue as a committed dyad and to make the process as smooth as possible. If A, B, and C co-own a home together, and if B and C will stay together, B and C may wish to retain the home, with A selling their one-third ownership to B and C—in addition to dividing up personal possessions.

Another question that needs to be decided is whether A will remain connected to B and/or C sexually on the secondary level, or as nonsexual friends, or not at all.

9.12

If two members of the triad (A and B) decide together that they no longer wish to continue in a primary triad relationship with C, then again, A and B should discuss the situation thoroughly with C, explaining to C why they (A and B) feel that they would like to be a twosome (or why they feel that having C as a primary partner is not a good fit for them), and whether either or both of them wish to continue sexually with C on the secondary level, or as nonsexual friends.

If there are children. What will become of children in the triad that is dissolving will depend on different factors, unrelated to whether one or two of the triad's partners initiate the breakup. Young children, of course, have no concept of biological parentage; for them, the essence of being a "mommy" or a "daddy" has to do 100% with their emotional connection to the adult in question, resulting in turn from their real-life interactions with that adult. Likewise, for a small enough child, a "brother" or "sister" is another kid who lives in your home with you (including "temporary siblings" such as foster children, exchange students, etc.).

The kinds of emotional connection that the child is likely to have with the adults and with other children in the home in turn depends on other factors. Was the child born into the triad family, or was the triad formed after the child was born and old enough to have formed child-parent and child-sibling bonds with one or more of the other people sharing the home?

Regardless of the time sequence, some multi-adult families cultivate a home atmosphere in which all adults are considered as equal "parents" of all the children, regardless of whose DNA is in which child. (Of course this is no different from two-parent homes with adopted or step children.) In other multi-adult families, a child knows (when they are old enough) which adult(s) are their "real" parents, although, again, all adults will typically interact in a parental way with all children in the household, helping them get dressed and go to bed, preparing meals, helping with homework, taking care of them in sickness, doing family outings together, and all the rest. This is discussed in more detail in section 9.06.

So when a multi-adult family with children breaks up, how are things handled for and with the children?

In households in which a child knows which are their "real" parent(s) and "real" sibling(s), and if after breakup the "real" parent(s) will continue with custody, things might be emotionally somewhat easier for the child than when one or more of a larger group of equal "parents" leaves, for their own reasons mysterious to the child. In any of those situations, however, the child will definitely experience a loss. Besides the "parents", if one or more *children* go one way and one or more go the other way, with their respective "real" parents, then each child is also losing siblings, not just parents. The child will go through a grieving period, and this should be recognized.

The adults should also be alert to the fact (as discussed in section 7.04) that children are easily and strongly molded by their experiences, for better or worse and with effects typically lasting indefinitely into adulthood unless, after the children grow into adults, they take measures to alleviate or nullify those associations. In other words, the formation of a triad or larger can form good, positive emotional associations for a child; the breakup of the triad (the same as the breakup of a dyad) could create future "hot buttons" later in life, with unfortunate consequences. Knowing this, when primary partners are contemplating dissolving a multi-adult family, and there are children in the home, special effort should be made to minimize the disruption, to keep the children informed to the extent of their maturity, and to assure them that they will not be abandoned but that they are still loved, they will still have a home with loving parents, and so on.

9.12

If (hopefully) the adults will continue to have some sort of ongoing interactions with each other, it would be good to make a special effort to include the children, at least occasionally, so the children can continue their own relationship with the departed adults and children to the extent possible.

~ 10 ~

Legalities

Contents:
10.01. Overview.
10.02. Living wills.
10.03. Powers of attorney.
10.04. Inheritance.
10.05. Owning real estate.
10.06. Parents and children.
10.07. Hassles and discrimination.
10.08. Zoning.
10.09. Child custody.
10.10. Libel, slander, and defamation of character.
10.11. Rights connected to marriage.

♥ ♥ ♥

10.01. Overview.

Legal concerns for poly people (as for anyone else) might be broadly divided into two categories—positive and negative, or active and passive. The positive and active concerns relate to things we want to do, or that we recognize are important to do, such as establishing living wills and testamentary wills, or owning real estate or other possessions jointly. The negative and passive ones involve legally defending an individual or family and standing up for our rights and freedoms when a bigoted, polyphobic government or individual attempts to take legal action against us, such as trying to evict us because of zoning, depriving us of legal custody of our children, or defaming our character, only because of our polyamorous lifestyle.

This chapter will deal with all these legal considerations.

This chapter is designed to offer general information and guidance; in no way can this chapter substitute for obtaining professional advice from an attorney. Furthermore, laws vary from place to place, and can change from time to time; and, as in other aspects of life, the fact of your polyamorous lifestyle can add complications to these legal situations. Therefore I strongly suggest that you consult an attorney even for seemingly straightforward matters such as preparing a living will, a durable power of attorney, a testamentary will, etc., even though "kits" are commonly available for these legal documents in office supply stores and elsewhere, and you can execute a legally valid document of these sorts without an attorney; generally all you need are witnesses and a notary public.

See the separate sections below for more detailed discussions.

10.02. Living wills.

Why they are needed. When an adult is unable to make normal decisions or do other intellectual functioning, or is unable to express their decisions and desires, because they are comatose, intellectually underdeveloped, severely mentally ill, or for other medical reasons, the law in every jurisdiction provides in various ways that someone else may make those decisions or take actions on the individual's behalf. In the specific case of someone who is terminally ill and comatose, the concept of the "living will" has been developed to allow an individual to let others know how they would like to be treated in that situation, while they are still in sound mental health, *before* the medical emergency arises.

In the absence of a living will (or sometimes even if there is one), local law also has procedures for a close relative to act on an incompetent person's behalf. As you might expect, however, no legal jurisdiction (at this writing) recognizes the standing of multiple primary partners for this process, which makes it all the more important, if you are in a multi-adult family, to have your wishes in this matter down in writing in a legally recognized form.

Unfortunately, even without the added complexity of multi-adult families, we occasionally hear in the news about a sad case of someone who has been lying comatose and in a vegetative state for a long time, their body supported by life-support apparatus (artificial nutrition, hydration, ventilation, kidney dialysis, etc.), with no hope of recovery, likewise no prospects of physical death as long as the life-support remains connected; and one close relative (say, the person's spouse) wants to withdraw life-support and allow the person (and the family!) a peaceful and dignified release and closure, but another relative (maybe a parent) insists on maintaining the state of limbo by continuing the mechanical life-support, thus creating a tragic and totally pointless legal battle and draining the family's assets for legal and medical costs on top of the emotional tragedy of the person's physical and mental condition.

What is a "living will"? A "living will" is a legal document that is designed to circumvent this sort of dilemma and tragedy, at least in many cases, by providing guidance and direction for the family and the healthcare providers in the eventuality that the person making the living will becomes unable to express their own desires about medical procedures, generally because the individual has become comatose or demented. A living will thus answers the question of "what they would want" if the comatose or demented person could only say so and sign a document. The signed document already exists.

10.02

See section 10.03 about powers of attorney, and the differences between a living will and a power of attorney.

Discuss with your primary partner(s). "Kits" are available inexpensively, with basic information and sample living will forms and other forms, from office supply stores and elsewhere. These can be very helpful in giving you broad information about the questions you want to consider, general legal requirements, etc. The legally required contents of a living will vary in detail from state to state, province to province; therefore you should consult an attorney in your jurisdiction.

However, before visiting an attorney, you should sit and talk with your primary partner(s) about the wishes of each of you in this and similar questions (organ donation, autopsy, disposal of the body after death, etc.). If you have bought a living will "kit", you can fill out the form which the kit says is appropriate for your jurisdiction, and take that to the attorney for them either to approve or to modify as necessary. It would be best *not* to sign the document before you visit the attorney, because the signing process (involving witnesses and a notary public, as described below) would have to be repeated if the attorney does advise changes.

A legally competent adult (that is, *any* person who has reached the local minimum age for adulthood, *unless* there has been some finding of legal *incompetence* due to mental illness or any other cause) draws up the living will, stating their wishes about whether to keep their body alive by artificial means when conscious brain functioning cannot return and there is no reasonable hope of recovery; and any other relevant questions.

Signing and witnessing. The form generally should be signed in the presence of two disinterested witnesses and of a notary public. A "disinterested" witness is one who would have no interest in the fact or timing of your death; thus, for example, someone that you name in your testamentary will to inherit something from you, or who would become entitled to a pension upon your death, should *not* be a witness to your living will. Any healthcare professional who might be involved in treating you also should not be a witness. Your attorney should be able to advise you more specifically about who would or would not be a suitable witness.

Are living wills honored by doctors and hospitals? Legal provisions about living wills vary in different states and provinces; most jurisdictions (at this writing) call for living wills to be honored. Some places require that a diagnosis of a terminal illness must be made *before* a living will is executed.

Generally, regardless of legal provisions, medical professionals honor living wills, and welcome them to help them decide how to treat their patients. (In the United States, the concept of living wills has been endorsed by both the American Medical Association—the professional association for physicians—and the American Hospital Association.)

Be aware, though, that even with a living will your wishes *may not* be honored. Nevertheless, it is far better to have one in place than not, because, if nothing else, a living will can help your closest loved ones negotiate with medical professionals and government officials about continuing or withholding ongoing artificial life support, based on "what you would want".

Although a living will requires some thought, discussion with your primary partner(s) and other family, and effort to execute, the "hassle" involved in preparing one is generally far less than the hassle and heartache that can ensue if you do not have one.

Guardianship. A court can appoint someone to act on behalf of a mentally incompetent adult, or on behalf of a minor if there is no one in the parental role to serve that function. However, you should not rely on the guardianship process to take the place of a living will or durable power of attorney (discussed in section 10.03), because (a) it could take weeks to months for the court to appoint a guardian; (b) the guardian chosen might not be someone you would want in that role; (c) attorney and court fees can be quite high, especially if the action is contested.

10.03. Powers of attorney.

What is a "power of attorney"? A "power of attorney", broadly speaking, is any document whereby you authorize someone else to make legally binding decisions and actions on your behalf while you are living.

A power of attorney does not require you to be comatose or otherwise mentally incompetent in order to go into effect; it is designed for more ordinary situations in which it is impossible or just inconvenient for you to act on your own behalf, and so you designate some trusted person to act for you. In fact, unless specified otherwise, a power of attorney ceases to have effect if you become medically unable to act on your own behalf (so in this sense it is exactly opposite to a living will—see section 10.02). You can, however, specify that a power of attorney is to remain in effect or go into effect if you become mentally incapacitated. This is called a "durable" power of attorney.

The person whom you designate in a power of attorney is called your "agent" or "attorney-in-fact". Do not be confused by the term "attorney-in-fact", because that person does not need to be an attorney *at law,* that is, a lawyer. Any legally competent person can serve as your "agent" or "attorney-in-fact". In this discussion I will use the simpler term "agent".

There are various types of power of attorney. As the name suggests, a "general" power of attorney is one in which you authorize another person (your agent) to take any action on your behalf, while in a "limited" power of attorney you specifically limit your agent's authority to one or more specific functions, for example, financial, business, or medical. You can have several limited powers of attorney in effect at the same time, as long as the specific functions of your agents do not overlap.

An example of "limited power of attorney" that many people are familiar with comes into play in buying and selling real estate. If the buyer or seller cannot be present at settlement, or simply does not wish to, they often give their realtor power of attorney to sign all the papers on their half.

A power of attorney can be open-ended in time, but typically you will specify a time period during which it is valid; or the power of attorney may be for a one-time action, such as voting in an organization's election or buying or selling a particular piece of real estate.

10.04. Inheritance.

The terminology. A "testamentary will", also formally called a "last will and testament", is what most people informally call simply a "will"—and that is the term that I will use here. This is the document in which you state who gets what possessions and assets of yours, and what is to become of your minor children and any incompetent adult dependents, upon your death.

In using the unmodified term "will", though, you need to be careful not to confuse this kind of will with a "living will" (described in section 10.02), which has a specific function while you are still living.

Why you need a will. As in the case of living but mentally incompetent persons (section 10.02), laws in every state or province provide for disposition of a deceased person's property, appointment of a guardian for minor children, etc., if there is no will. However, if you die without a will ("to die intestate" is the legal term), your assets quite likely will not be transferred the way you would like, and the person appointed to oversee the process may not be someone you would choose. A will can let you specify exactly who gets what and who should look after your children, etc., as well as who is to see to it that your will is honored.

Repeating the refrain one more time, the added complications of polyamory, especially multi-adult families, make it all the more important for you to specify your exact wishes in a formal will. If you have multiple primary partners whom you want to inherit, or if you want to bequeath something to a secondary partner, you can do this in a will; without a will, it probably will not happen.

Likewise, you can specify your primary partners in sequence as guardians for your children (see below in this section). Otherwise, your children might well be uprooted from their familiar home (in addition to the trauma of your death) and sent to live with their grandparents, an aunt and uncle, etc.

If you are in a committed dyad or in a multi-adult family, you and your primary partner(s) can (if you wish) make "reciprocal" wills, essentially identical but naming each other as beneficiaries, guardian of children, etc.

As is true for living wills, "kits" for testamentary wills are available inexpensively, with basic information and sample will forms and other forms, from office supply stores and elsewhere.

Modifying a will. A will can be modified by attaching an amendment, called a "codicil", to the original will. The codicil must be signed and witnessed in the same manner (but not necessarily by the same people) as the original will. Another method, of course, is to establish a completely new will that revokes and replaces the previous one.

You should consider revising your will or replacing it with a new one if you have a new child or a child reaches maturity, if you divorce or separate, or if you add one or more new primary partners. Marriage automatically cancels any existing will, and so you *must* establish a new will after getting married. You may also want to consider revising or replacing your will if your financial situation changes substantially, since you may wish to change how to dispose of your assets.

There can be many other reasons for revising or replacing a will, especially for the polyamorous person, as personal circumstances change. The general consensus is that you should review your will at least once a year to see if you need to make any updates.

What the will contains. There are standard items that any will should include.

The first is to name your "personal representative", or "executor", and at least one alternate. This is the person who will work with the court to see that your will is carried out as you specified.

Second, if you have minor children or any incompetent adult dependents, name someone to serve as guardian. Only one person can be guardian at a time, but you should name one or more alternates in case the first named person is unable or unwilling to serve.

Typically, your primary partner, or one of them, would be named as guardian—someone who is already closely involved with your children and who would be willing to continue caring for your children and any other dependents if you die. If you have multiple primary partners, it is especially important to list each of them (if that is your wish) in some order as alternate guardians, because, if your family remains intact after your death, only in this way can you be reasonably assured that your children will be able to remain in their familiar home with the ones they know and love in the parental role.

Third, your will should describe any specific bequests. This can be a certain object or collection that you would like someone in particular to have for sentimental or other reasons; or a specified sum of money, stock certificates, etc., that you wish to leave to a particular person or organization. Name a contingency beneficiary in case the first person named dies before you.

Fourth, as a "catch-all", designate who gets everything remaining after the specific bequests have been honored. If you do not wish to make any specific bequests, then you can simply state that you leave everything to a particular person or category of persons, such as your primary partners and/or your children. You should name one or more contingency beneficiaries in case the person(s) you name first die before you do.

Name each person by name and relationship, rather than just saying "to all my children" or "to all my partners", for example. This is especially important, of course, if you are designating plural primary partners as a group of beneficiaries in this category (since at this writing such a concept is unknown to the law), or if you are in a multi-adult, multi-child family and you are bequeathing part or all of your assets to the children in the family, who may be of various biological and legal parentage.

You also need to specify what happens if one or more of your named beneficiaries die before you do. Let's suppose you are in a quad, you bequeath everything to your three primary partners, and one of your primaries dies before you do. Do the two surviving partners divide everything two ways, or do the legal *survivors* (usually children) of your *deceased* partner get a one-third share, further divided among them? State your preference.

You can sometimes specifically *exclude* someone from the "catch-all" category of beneficiaries—say, one of your children or a legal spouse—but there are limitations on this in some jurisdictions. If you do exclude someone, you should not just refrain from naming them as a beneficiary, but explicitly state that you are excluding someone that you name, their relationship to you, and why (for example, your grown daughter Mary because of lack of contact with her for many years).

In your will you can also, if you wish, cancel any cash debts that anyone may owe you. You should be specific on this point if you have given money to someone (such as a grown child), say for college expenses or to help them buy a car or a home, and if that person will also be a beneficiary of part of your assets. Do you consider the money provided to be a loan or an outright gift? If a loan, should the unpaid balance be deducted from what they would otherwise inherit, or are you writing the loan off before your assets are dispersed?

Signing and witnessing. As with living wills (see section 10.02), a testamentary will must be signed in the presence of two disinterested witnesses and a notary public. A "disinterested" witness in this case is someone who would have no interest in the matters discussed in the will; that is, they are not named as a beneficiary, nor named as executor or guardian, or alternate. Your attorney should be able to advise you about who would or would not be a "disinterested" witness.

As mentioned in section 10.01, I highly recommend consulting an attorney, especially for the more complicated family arrangements that polyamory can entail. Do not sign the will before consulting the attorney, because if the attorney recommends any changes, you will then need to trouble your witnesses to go through the signing process again.

Related matters. In addition to the will itself, it is a good idea to prepare statements and lists of information that your family would need if you die. This includes, of course, where the will (and other important documents) are located. You can specify your wishes about things like whether you prefer cremation or burial. (Another option is to have your body donated to a medical college, since medical students must learn anatomy by dissecting cadavers.) Do you have a preference as to where you would like to be buried, or whether or where to have your ashes scattered?

You can also list life insurance policies, bank accounts, stocks, and pension information, with account numbers, and where the relevant papers are stored.

Only the signed original of a will (or living will or similar document) is legally valid, but it can be helpful to the survivors to have one or more photocopies of your will (etc.) readily available for planning and informational purposes. A photocopy will also help you review your will periodically, as mentioned above, so you can decide if you want to make any updates.

10.05. *Owning real estate.*

The news here is generally good—that is, that generally there are no obstacles to purchasing real estate in the name of more than two parties. I myself have done it twice: When my first wife and I formed a quad with another couple, the four of us bought a house together and lived in it. More recently, when my two primaries and I were attempting to form a triad, we bought a house together that would have been our shared home (but we decided not to continue as a triad before we actually moved in together). All that's required is to let the real estate agent or other parties know how many are making the purchase, and their names, so that the transfer documents can be prepared showing the right names and right number of spaces for signatures.

If you will be obtaining a mortgage in order to finance the purchase, that is a separate legal transaction from the actual purchase. If you will be depending on the income and assets of two or more of you in order to secure the mortgage, let the bank or credit union know this when you apply for your mortgage.

Zoning is an entirely different matter. If you are a triad or larger, you would be wise to check the zoning provisions of any home you are contemplating buying or renting. If it is zoned for a maximum of two adults, you might face legal opposition to your living there. If it is zoned for "single family" occupancy, of course you can argue (if it comes to that) that the three or four of you, etc., do constitute one single family—but you might have to face your local zoning authority or public prosecuting official refusing to recognize the validity of a polyamorous multi-adult family.

So if there is some question about zoning that the zoning authority cannot answer to your satisfaction, decide, before you buy or rent a home, if you would be willing to carry through with that kind of court battle, with uncertain outcome.

See section 10.07 about hassles and discrimination, including zoning disputes. See section 10.08 for a more general discussion of zoning with regard to multi-adult families.

10.06. *Parents and children.*

Permissions and other actions on behalf of a child. Section 9.06 discusses how the adults in a multi-adult family could interact with the children, one option being that all the adults coequally identify as parents for all the children, regardless of biological or legal parent-child status. However, even if your family functions smoothly this way day to day, there are times when only a *legally recognized* parent may act in the parental role. These situations involve such things as a parent signing a permission slip for a class trip or activity at the child's school, or giving permission for some medical treatment or test.

This is usually not a problem in a typical multi-adult family, in which at least one of the adults in the family does have that legal status as parent, either by being the biological or adoptive parent of the child or by having a step-parent relationship through marriage. In these cases, a legal parent in the family can sign the permission form etc.

There is little point in deliberately making an issue of the parental role of another adult in the family, by insisting that the signature of the other adult be honored. My hunch is that if such a case were to be taken to court, any judge would rule that there is no reason why the legal parent in the household could not and should not sign the form on the child's behalf.

In the unusual case in which a child for some reason is living in a household in which none of the adults have the status of legal parent or guardian, probably the family should arrange to have one of the adults appointed as guardian for the child. In that case, of course, the guardian would be legally entitled to sign such permission forms.

Another situation in which the *legal* parent-child status is relevant is for insurance and pensions. For example, under the Social Security (social insurance) system in the United States, a minor child (or student, through college to age 22) of an insured worker becomes entitled to monthly cash benefits if the worker/parent dies or becomes entitled to retirement or disability benefits; and the child's other legal parent may also be entitled.

Custody and child support. Certainly poly families are susceptible to separations as are traditional dyadic families. Disputes sometimes arise as to who will have legal custody of a child of that family following separation, and the noncustodial parent is often asked to make child support payments.

Again, only a *legal* parent may normally request a court for custody, and only a *legal* noncustodial parent can be obligated to pay child support. (Custody is sometimes assigned to someone other than a legal parent, even if a parent is available, if the court deems that to be in the child's best interest. Whenever possible this is another close relative, such as an aunt, uncle, or grandparent. Sometimes a court will assign joint or shared custody.)

This can raise the question as to *who is* a legal parent in the case of a child born into a multi-adult family containing two or more men, if the family is uncertain who is the biological father of the child.

Also see section 10.09 about attempts by outsiders to deprive your family of custody of a child due to nothing more than your polyamorous lifestyle.

Determining biological parentage. Even if the family treats all adult family members as having an equal parental role, and does not care which man is the biological father of a given child, the situations discussed above can make it necessary to know who is the biological father. As section 9.06 notes, there can be other (nonlegal) reasons for wanting to know biological parentage, for example if a (possible) parent or grandparent or other relative of the child is diagnosed with a heritable disease.

For these reasons it is a good idea to have biological parentage routinely determined by testing, reasonably promptly after a child's birth, if parentage is not readily known and agreed by all male partners in the family. This should not be thought of as contentious but just anticipating future problems, similar to taking out an insurance policy or making a will.

10.07. Hassles and discrimination.

What underlies bigotry. There seems to be an urge deep in many people's psyches (I don't think it's part of the hard-wired human subconscious) to look down on other people who are different in some way—ethnicity, religion, lifestyle, you name it. This is probably rooted in the twin psychological phenomena of low self-esteem and projection—"projection" being the unconscious tendency to attribute to others negative feelings about oneself that one is psychologically unable to acknowledge consciously. For example, if I am unable to admit my own boorishness, lack of intelligence, lack of ethics, etc., then it's those other guys over there who are uncouth, stupid, immoral, etc., not *me*.

Unfortunately, this tendency gets reinforced by another bit of mental sloppiness, the belief that something is more likely to be true, the more people claim it to be true. So for example (this "reasoning" goes), if most people in my society believe that people from Bloopdedoopia are lazy, then it must be true, and therefore this Bloopdedoopian that we see there is lazy. "My mind's made up, so don't confuse me with the facts." Of course this sort of herd thinking just reinforces itself.

When discrimination and bigotry is by government itself. Going one step further, all governments tend to reflect popular prejudices, reflecting the prejudices or bigotry of those people who constitute the government. When bigotry or prejudice becomes embedded in official government policy, it manifests as discrimination.

Many nominally democratic governments have adopted lofty legal principles protecting personal freedoms and minority rights, but the reality often doesn't match the ideal. Otherwise there never would have been a need for Mahatma Gandhi, Susan B. Anthony, César Chávez, Martin Luther King, Jr., Nelson Mandela, and many others. Still, it's always better to have these principles in place than not, as a legal grounds on which to base court challenges of unfair treatment, either by individuals or by the government.

Being on the receiving end of bigotry is never easy, whether your government officially sides with you or with the herd-thinkers. As of this writing, I have not yet seen much bigotry directed toward the polyamory community—but that may just be because we have not become very visible yet; we're "under the radar". Also, to the extent that we *are* visible, we haven't been very noisy yet in asserting rights and privileges for poly families. Alas, if the experience of gays and lesbians in the United States is any indicator, we may well start drawing flak when more of us do start coming out of the closet, when more people identify as poly because it's better known, when more books on the theme of polyamory are on the market, when talk show hosts invite more poly guests, and so on.

Strength in numbers. The good news in the above is that the same greater numbers that give us visibility and bring flak upon us also give us the strength to insist on fair treatment, both through official channels such as legislation and the courts and through the well used and effective channels of public persuasion such as letter-writing campaigns, petitions, public demonstrations, and just getting to know our nonpoly neighbors and associates and becoming friends with them, showing them that we are decent, ethical people.

In this section we've talked about general, unfocused ways in which individuals or the poly community as a whole might receive unfair, bigoted treatment, and how we might respond. In sections 10.08, 10.09, and 10.10 we will look at a few specific ways in which the bigotry and discrimination might be directed at us.

10.08. Zoning.

Most or all areas with some density of human presence have been divided up into zones according to what the land may legally be used for. Mostly this is a good thing, so that, for example, if you move into a nice house with room for a vegetable garden and grass for your kids to play on, you won't find a smelly and toxic chemical plant being built next door to you a year later.

Residential zoning can be further subdivided into a maximum of two adults per household, or a single family per household, or larger numbers (among other categories, such as single-family residences or multi-unit apartment or condominium buildings). The latter might, for example, allow a residence for the elderly—or that might be a zoning category of its own.

Polyamorous multi-adult families can run into problems with zoning, because when three of us share one bed, or if we use two or more bedrooms in a larger house, we are typically in the market for the same kind of housing as are dyadic or single-adult households, especially families consisting of two parents and several children. These homes are, of course, the ones most likely to be zoned either for two adults or for a "single family".

At least as of this writing, zoning problems for multi-adult poly families are probably not *deliberately* the result of attempts to keep poly families out of the neighborhood; it's just that the assumption has been all along that if there are more than two adults, it must be more than one "family". The worthy intention is to avoid overcrowding.

This may be a future political campaign for the poly community—either to get officialdom to acknowledge the "single family" concept to include triads, quads, etc., or to get new categories of zoning enacted that envision multi-adult families.

As mentioned in section 10.05, any multi-adult family should check the specific wording of the zoning applicable to a given residence before they buy it or sign a rental lease, to ensure that they are not walking into a legal battle and/or the tragedy and financial loss of not being able to live there all together. The same also applies before a third adult moves into a two-adult household.

10.09. *Child custody.*

In addition to the internal disputes about child custody that sometimes arise when parents separate, the poly community has already seen at least one case in which a woman whose grown daughter was in a triad with two men and who believed that a multi-adult family was inherently immoral and an unfit environment for her granddaughter (the younger woman's toddler-age daughter), sued to deprive the three loving parents of custody of the child—and the judge agreed (in spite of expert witnesses supporting the healthiness of the triad's home environment, who were ignored) and pulled the child from the home, giving custody to the grandmother.

It is easy to analyze situations like that in hindsight, after the damage is done, but hard to repair the damage. In that case, the woman in the triad had appeared with her two partners on a local TV program, the grandmother saw the program, and that's how the grandmother came to learn of the triad. It occurred in the southeastern United States, not noted for an enlightened judiciary or other branches of government (not that we can trust the judiciary or other branches of government elsewhere, come to that).

We can, however, learn lessons from these events that can improve our wisdom for other similar situations in the future.

We need to stay informed about how enlightened our legislatures, courts, and administrative branches of government all are—how likely they are to treat us fairly or with anti-polyamory bigotry. We need to be careful of our own behavior—which does not mean caving in to the bigots, but it does mean using common sense about when or how we let our lifestyle be seen in the general community.

There's nothing wrong with taking risks, but we should *consciously* weigh risks and benefits. We need to think *consciously* about what risks we are taking, to ourselves or to our children, by letting our polyamory be visible, either small-scale, as by walking down a street hand-in-hand-in-hand, or massively (even if only on the local scale) by letting our multi-adult family appear on television.

10.10. Libel, slander, and defamation of character.

To "defame" someone is to knowingly make a false statement about that person publicly that damages their reputation. "False" can be either untrue or not established as true. "Defamation of character" is one of those needlessly and unnecessarily redundant and duplicative courtly and judicial terms and phrases that use and utilize three or more words or locutions when one would do nicely. But if someone says nasty, untrue things about you because of your polyamorous lifestyle (or for whatever reason), "defamation of character" is what you want to call it when you go to talk with your lawyer about possibly suing for damages.

If a defamatory statement is in writing (say in a newspaper, a blog, a book, or any other publicly distributed written material), it is legally called "libel". If it is oral (on a radio or TV news program or talk show, for example, or someone giving a talk at a public rally), it is "slander". Thus, "libel" and "slander" are subcategories of "defamation", and so your suit for damages may mention "libel" or "slander" rather than "defamation of character".

Suppose your local newspaper printed a story that started like this: "A gunman yesterday shot and killed someone in a parking lot here in Ourtown. Police quickly captured the murderer, Joe Blow, of 123 First Avenue, Ourtown." Joe Blow could immediately sue the newspaper for libel, and he would win, no matter how many unimpeachable eyewitnesses identified him to police as the fellow who pulled the trigger. The reason is that under the legal system in the United States (and I think this principle must be fairly general in the world), Joe Blow is presumed innocent of any crime until proven guilty in court or by other established legal process, no matter how strong the evidence against him appears to be. Calling him a "murderer" *before* a jury brings a conviction, if they do, thus defames him.

This is why the word "alleged" is so commonly used in our "news" media, which are so fond of emphasizing violent, barbaric events in our society, such as murder cases, and ignoring the truly important positive news going on all around us. If the newspaper had said, "Police quickly captured the alleged murderer, Joe Blow…," or "Police quickly captured Joe Blow, whom bystanders identified as the gunman …," now Joe Blow has no libel case, because it is a verifiable fact that police are *alleging* that Joe Blow did the deed and is being charged with murder, and fact that the bystanders made their statements to the police about the gunman's identity. If Joe Blow is later convicted of murder, and all his appeals are to no avail, then it is proper to refer publicly to "murderer Joe Blow".

If someone says or writes something nasty about you, due to polyphobia or any other reason, by all means be ready to stand up for your rights and seek redress in court if that seems appropriate, and worth the effort and cost to you. Just keep in mind each of the requirements under law for the nasty remark to qualify as "defamation", "libel", or "slander". It must be public, so that an insult to you in your living room or on the phone does not count. It has to be untrue, or unverified, so (let's say) if you *really are* behind on your child support payments, you can't sue a newspaper for libel or defamation of character if it publicizes that fact. The statement must also be something that reasonably would damage your reputation among other people.

10.11. Rights connected to marriage.

"Marriage" is a strictly *legal* concept, even though marriage ceremonies have been conducted by clergy of every organized religious variety probably far longer than civil officials have been empowered to solemnize marriage. The reason why marriage is legal, not religious, is that it is the *laws* in a given jurisdiction, and *only* those laws, that determine who may marry, or which marriage ceremonies will be recognized as valid. Clergy may conduct a lovely ceremony and end with some words like "I now pronounce you husband and wife," or "I now pronounce that you are married partners together," but unless the local *law* recognizes the particular human combination in which the partners fit as being eligible to marry each other (and the government has to issue a "marriage license", which attests to eligibility), and no matter how many well-wishers attend the ceremony and eat and dance at the reception afterwards, they aren't married.

Not only that, but the only real-life consequences of marriage are *legal privileges and responsibilities,* such as cheaper taxes, entitlement to pensions and insurance, inheritance by a surviving spouse or children, support obligations, the right to act on behalf of someone mentally unable to manage their own affairs, the right to visit someone in the hospital, and the like.

Among gays and lesbians, a ceremony that looks like a wedding but usually has no *legal* status is commonly called a "commitment ceremony". It is just as lovely as a legally valid wedding, because the *personal and social* significance is in the public declaration by the partners of their mutual commitment, embedded in other beautiful words and beautiful music, perhaps presided over by a clergy—someone whose profession has to do with the most significant interactions that we humans have with each other and with higher levels of consciousness.

We in the polyamory community can have "commitment ceremonies" also, if we wish, presided over by clergy, including ceremonies for three or more partners. As with gays and lesbians, these pretty ceremonies will have no *legal* effect unless or until some day we obtain legal recognition of our multi-adult families.

The campaign among gays and lesbians to gain the right to marry (that is, to gain those basic civil rights partially listed in the second paragraph above), as of this writing, is starting to take root in statutory and case law, but still has a long way to go. The possibility of polyamorous marriage, that is, marriage of more than two people together, at this writing is not even a glimmer beyond the horizon. It is rarely mentioned currently even within the polyamory community. Whether future generations of polyamorists will want to work to gain the right to marry in numbers larger than two at a time is something that only the future will reveal.

~ Appendix A ~

Resources

Contents:
A.01. Overview.
A.02. Therapists and attorneys.
A.03. Global, national, and electronic organizations.
A.04. Regional and local organizations.
A.05. Books.
A.06. Sexual hygiene.

♥ ♥ ♥

A.01. Overview.

This appendix contains references to organizations, websites, other books, and other resources that you may find helpful.

All sections of this appendix are likely to be incomplete, some websites no longer functional, etc., simply because of the rapid evolution of new sites and organizations, publication of new books, etc. I apologize if your site, your organization, your book, etc., is not listed here, or shows the wrong information. Please see the paragraph of the introduction headed "Your input is invited" (page xxii) about how you can help this information be more up-to-date for the next edition of this work.

A.02. Therapists and attorneys.

On email groups maintained by local poly organizations, people sometimes ask for references to psychotherapists, healers, or attorneys known to be "poly-friendly".

Appendix A

Of course it would be impractical to include in this appendix a comprehensive listing of known poly-friendly therapists and attorneys in all areas, both because of the size of the list and because many worthy practitioners would be left out.

There is, however, one online group of professional counselors intentionally set up to address this need for sympathetic, aware counselors, and that's Kink Aware Professionals. If you don't think of your sexual habits as "kinky" (you like "vanilla" sex, only two at a time, with loving foreplay, followed by Tab A in Slot B, and so on), don't be put off by the word "kink" in the name of this organization. Yes, they are also there for people into BDSM, fetishes, or other sexual minorities; but they certainly will be sympathetic to polyamory, regardless of how tame or adventurous is your own sexual expression.

Their website is http://www.ncsfreedom.org/index.php?option=com_keyword&id=270—which is actually a subpage of the National Coalition for Sexual Freedom, another worthwhile organization; see section A.03.

One way to get a referral is to post your request to a local poly email group. Some local poly groups may maintain their own lists of known local friendly professionals. (See section A.04 for information about locating local poly groups.)

We should also note two particular *categories* of professional personal counselors who, as a group, stand out as being understanding and accepting of alternative lifestyles in general, who are (generally speaking) not in the least narrow-minded or judgmental, and who are fully capable of offering competent personal counseling. Many of them participate in one or another alternative lifestyle themselves. Those groups are Pagan priests and priestesses, and Unitarian clergy (Unitarian-Universalist in the United States).

Appendix A

Of course you do not need to follow either of those particular spiritual paths yourself (or style of paths, or any path, for that matter) to be welcomed into either a Pagan priest's or priestess's or Unitarian minister's office, and both Pagans and Unitarians (clergy and lay members equally) are scrupulously opposed to dogma and proselytizing, so you can make an appointment with any of these with full assurance that you will not find yourself on the receiving end of a sales pitch for Paganism or Unitarianism, regardless of your own spiritual views or lack thereof.

If your particular situation truly requires the expertise of a psychotherapist or psychiatrist, a Pagan priest or priestess or a Unitarian minister in your area quite likely will be able to refer you to someone known to be accepting and not judgmental or biased against alternative lifestyles or orientations; or see section A.03, the entry for the National Coalition for Sexual Freedom.

The clergy or leaders of other progressive or liberal religious traditions, such as Reform Judaism and the Society of Friends (Quakers), may also be sympathetic toward polyamory.

Section 7.14 refers to spiritual or energetic healing as a sometimes very fast and effective alternative to psychotherapy. As noted there, one problem with this is to locate someone with genuine skills to do this healing, since there is not yet any accreditation process, so that anyone regardless of competence can hang out a shingle.

There is one reliable referral source known to the author for spiritual healing. That is Renaissance of the Heart, LLC, www.HeartHealing.net.

One convenient feature of spiritual healing, in contrast to psychotherapy, is that spiritual healing does not require physical proximity. A competent healer will be able to see or otherwise sense your situation, and heal it, regardless of how far apart you and the healer

Appendix A

are geographically, and so healers typically work by phone as well as in person for those who happen to be nearby.

For conventional psychotherapeutic counseling, you may wish to ask your local poly group or email list, or your physician, for suggestions. You can also look under "Counselors" in the yellow pages phone book.

A.03. Global, national, and electronic organizations.

Loving More: POB 4358 / Boulder, CO 80306-4358 / U.S.A.; 303-543-7540; www.lovemore.com; lovingmore@lovemore.com. Loving More is an umbrella poly organization in the U.S. that provides a number of services on their website, publishes a magazine, hosts a chatroom, and conducts annual conferences both in the western and the eastern U.S.

National Coalition for Sexual Freedom, www.ncsfreedom.org/index.php. This is an organization which (quoting from their website), "is a national organization committed to creating a political, legal, and social environment in the United States that advances equal rights of consenting adults who practice forms of alternative sexual expression. NCSF is primarily focused on the rights of consenting adults in the SM-leather-fetish, swing, and polyamory communities, who often face discrimination because of their sexual expression."

That pretty well sums it up: They are a proactive organization working for networking and freedom from discrimination or legal hassles because of any form of consensual adult sexual expression.

They also sponsor (as a subpage to their website) the Kink Awareness Professionals, a listing of professional psychotherapeutic counselors who are known to be sympathetic not just to polyamory but to any "alternative" or "minority" form of sexual or emotional relationship, including homosexual, BDSM, fetishistic, etc. See section A.02.

Appendix A

Bisexual Resource Center, The: http://www.biresource.org. As the name suggests, this is an online resource center offering information, contacts, books, conferences, etc., about bisexuality.

Fellowship for Intentional Community, http://www.ic.org/; 660-883-5545; RR 1 Box 156-W, Rutledge MO 63563-9720, USA. An active umbrella organization for the intentional community (IC) movement, offering many services, such as a directory of existing intentional communities, a magazine, conferences, books, a search service for ICs seeking members and individuals seeking ICs, etc.

Hendricks Institute, The: 400 W. Ojai Ave. / Suite 101, PMB 413 / Ojai, CA 93023 / U.S.A.; 800-688-0772; www.hendricks.com. This institute is led by Gay Hendricks, Ph.D., and Kathlyn Hendricks, Ph.D., coauthors of the book *Conscious Loving: The Journey to Co-Commitment,* listed in section A.05. The institute offers many seminars, programs, and other books designed to help people become more aware of the (often unconscious) dynamics going on in their interpersonal relationships.

Platinum Rule, The: www.platinumrule.com. This site is associated with the book by the same name by Tony Alessandra (listed under section A.05). Among other things, this site contains a self-administered test to let you decide which of four personality types you fit into, as described in more detail in the book.

Polyamory Chatroom: http://www.polyamorychat.com/.

Polyamory Society, The: http://www.polyamorysociety.org. An online organization providing information about polyamory, events, etc.; personal ads; chatroom and other services.

Polyamory Weekly: http://polyweekly.com/. An online series of podcasts and articles.

Polycamp NW: http://www.polycamp.org/. This site is for a loosely organized camping weekend for polys held annually in August in

Appendix A

northwestern Washington State. (A number of other "polycamps" also exist in other regions of North America, hosted by local poly groups. See also the next listing.)

Polycamp WV: http://www.polycamp.net/. This site is for a loosely organized camping weekend for polys held annually in August in West Virginia. (See also the preceding listing.)

Poly Event Search: http://www.polyliving.com/events. A search engine for poly events within a time frame and a geographical region that you specify.

PolyFamilies CampCon: http://www.polyfamilies.com/polycampcon.html. An annual poly family camping event in Vermont; the site also provides other services.

Poly Matchmaker: http://polymatchmaker.com/pmm3/main.mv?Screen=HTML&Page=membershipinfo. Primarily a poly-focused personal ad site, but also providing a book store, articles, and other services.

PolyOz: http://polyoz.dhs.org/. A poly organization serving Australia.

Unitarian-Universalists for Polyamory Awareness (UUPA): http://www.uupa.org. An organization affiliated with the Unitarian-Universalist Association, the national organization for this denomination in the United States. UUPA is for polyamorous Unitarian-Universalists.

World Polyamory Association (WPA): http://www.worldpolyamoryassociation.com/home2.html. In spite of the name, this organization is based in the United States and is focused on U.S. events. The email list does, however, attract postings occasionally from elsewhere in the world. WPA also provides a store, information, links, etc.

A.04. Regional and local organizations.

A list of local poly organizations and groups would tend to become outdated fairly quickly in a book, so no attempt is made here to include such a list. Loving More (see entry under section A.03) provides online links to local groups in the United States. For other parts of the world, try your local national or regional organization if one exists. If not, this is your opportunity to found a group! That's easier to do than you might think. See section 8.10.

A.05. Books.

I have found some of the following books especially enlightening and helpful in some aspect of the fundamental concepts that underlie what we have been talking about in this book (the dynamics of poly living), such as individual consciousness and attitudes and interpersonal communications and dynamics. Other books listed here are at least useful and worthwhile. In addition to the bare facts of author and publication data, I offer a personal comment on some of these books.

> Anapol, Deborah M., Ph.D. (1997). *Polyamory: The New Love Without Limits.* San Rafael, CA: IntiNet Resource Center. This is probably the first book published during the current awakening of the general polyamory community, and is still one of the best known. As a pioneer in the field, it focuses largely on what polyamory is, describing many of its characteristics.
>
> Anderlini-D'Onofrio, Serena, Ph.D., editor (2004). *Plural Loves: Designs for Bi and Poly Living.* Binghamton, NY: Harrington Park Press. This is a collection of articles, autobiographical accounts, fiction, etc., with the general theme of bisexuality and polyamory.
>
> Blanton, Brad (third edition, 2003). *Radical Honesty: How to Transform Your Life By Telling the Truth.* Stanley, Virginia: Sparrowhawk Publications. This is an important, groundbreaking exposé of how everyone is acculturated toward hiding the truth

from themselves as well as from others, and of the importance to personal and societal mental health of learning to be fully truthful (again, both in our self-acknowledgments and in what we communicate to others). Although the author does not comment on polyamory specifically, the principles he discusses are fundamental both to poly living and to many other aspects of life.

Christian, Diana Leafe. *Creating a Life Together* (2003) and *Finding Community* (2007). Both published by New Society Publishers, POB 189, Gabriola Island, BC V0R 1X0, Canada; www.newsociety.com. These two books are about joining and living in intentional communities (ICs). As section 2.07 notes, there are many similarities in the interpersonal dynamics between polyamory and life in an IC; indeed, polyamory is far more common in ICs than in the population as a whole, though polyamory is by no means universal in ICs. Because of the overlap of dynamics, these two books are especially useful to polyamorous and nonpoly people considering joining or forming an IC, but would also be very helpful to poly people with no specific interest in ICs.

Constantine, Larry and Joan (1973). *Group Marriage: A Study of Contemporary Multilateral Marriage.* New York, NY: The MacMillan Company. This work stands out as a rare beacon at its time, a generation before the word "polyamory" was coined, offering a sociological study of multi-adult committed relationships.

Hendricks, Gay, Ph.D., and Kathlyn Hendricks, Ph.D. (1990). *Conscious Loving: The Journey to Co-Commitment.* New York: Bantam Books. While the book speaks mostly of the dynamics between partners of a couple, the principles described here are very applicable as well to triads or larger committed groups. The authors, a couple who are themselves two psychotherapists, very clearly describe processes of openness and honesty between committed partners, and how even intelligent, enlightened people can overlook (not be open to) negative processes going on within their own psyches and in the couple dynamics. Highly recommended reading not only if you are having relationship problems but if things are okay for you and you want to make your relationship even better. Also see "The Hendricks Institute" under section A.03.

Kaldera, Raven (2005). *Pagan Polyamory.* Llewellyn Publications, Woodbury, Minnesota; www.llewellyn.com. As the title suggests, this work is aimed primarily at those in the Pagan community who are wondering about polyamory, as well as polyamorists who have a Pagan spiritual path of one sort or another. For example, there is discussion of love spells, and a handfasting ritual. However, there is also plenty of good wisdom here about polyamory in general, so if Paganism is not your spiritual path, do not be turned off by the word "Pagan" in the title.

McFetridge, Grant (with contributions from three co-authors) (2004). *Peak States of Consciousness, Volume 1.* Institute for the Study of Peak States, Hornby Island, British Columbia, Canada; www.peakstates.com. (Volumes 2 and 3 in this series, not yet published as of this writing, are projected to go into greater detail of the principles and processes, relevant especially for professional counselors and healers but useful also for lay persons, as Volume 1 also is.) This is a fascinating work describing groundbreaking research and discoveries, based on solid scientific principles and practices, that can quickly and simply lead people with "ordinary, normal" consciousness or awareness to achieve greatly enhanced states of consciousness and abilities at perception and healing, such as is usually associated only with a few people who have an especially enlightened level of spiritual development. Because polyamorous relationships tend to bring to light much material previously buried in unconscious levels of our psyches, the techniques in this book would be extremely valuable for processing that material and healing individuals of traumas and issues so that they can more smoothly lead a polyamorous life, along with any other aspect of life.

Tannen, Deborah (1990). *You Just Don't Understand: Women and Men in Conversation.* New York: William Morrow and Company, Inc. This book is a highly insightful and clear description of the typical differences, whether innate or culturally imprinted on us, in how women and men tend to express themselves—differences which, when not understood, often lead to annoying to tragic miscommunication between women and men. Highly recommended especially because of the high importance of effective and thorough communication in polyamory, regardless of gender.

A.06. Sexual hygiene.

The following are telephone numbers (all in the United States) connecting you to resources pertaining to sexual hygiene or sexually transmitted diseases. In the United States and probably other countries, you can also call your local public health department or local office of Planned Parenthood.

Appendix A

National STD Hotline: 800-321-4407.

National STD Hotline operated by the United States Center for Disease Control (CDC, an agency of the U.S. federal government): 800-227-8922.

National AIDS Hotline operated by the American Social Health Association: 800-342-AIDS.

National Herpes Hotline: 919-361-8488.

~ *Appendix B* ~
Glossary

A number of specialized terms are used in polyamory, and some ordinary words sometimes take on special meanings in a polyamorous context (e.g., "cheat", "faithful", "partner", "primary", "secondary"). Language is constantly evolving, and is always only an approximate expression of our thoughts and feelings at best. However, good communication is even more important in the poly world than elsewhere, and so we need to be especially vigilant about how we use words, especially new words that aren't in the dictionary, or words that we use in a way different from the standard dictionary definitions.

To help in this regard, I offer this Glossary of Terms, with my best effort at defining these terms as they are usually used within the context of polyamory and/or other nonmainstream forms of sexual relationships. Along with these definitions I also offer other commentary that I hope will shed some light on a word's origin or how it is used. Pronunciation guidance is offered for those few terms not currently found (with different definitions) in standard dictionaries.

Keep in mind, though, that there is no final authority for the definition of any given word, and polyamorous people (like everyone else) do use these words (like all other words) with variations of meaning. (One sometimes hears polyamorous people say that there are as many different definitions of the word "polyamory" as there are polyamorous people.)

Appendix B

In addition to the need to keep up with new terms and new definitions, accurate and complete communication becomes exponentially more important as the number of intimate partners rises from two to three or four or more, because the relationships become exponentially more complex. (Although Chapter 6 deals with relationship skills more broadly, verbal communication skills comprise a major part of that chapter.)

For these reasons it is especially important, when communicating with your partner(s) or any polyamorous person (as well as anyone else), to get clear with each other about just how each of *you* is using a given term, if there is any hint of ambiguity or possible miscommunication. Check the meaning given in this Glossary—but remember that this is just a starting point and a guide; what matters most to you and your partners is what *each of you* means by a given term, the notion that you each are symbolizing by the term. It will simplify matters greatly for you all if you can agree among yourselves about what a term means *for your partnership or group*.

Most of the terms in this glossary are either new terms, or entail new usages, that have arisen with polyamory as an identified modern social phenomenon (i.e., since about 1990). Some older terms are included when these are relevant, for example if they serve as a comparison to terms in polyamory, or if they have a new usage within the poly context. I am also including some terms that refer to relationships and sexuality in general, or to other ways of sexually relating, since these terms sometimes arise also in conversations and discussions among polys.

This glossary does *not* include the names of specific sexually transmitted diseases (STDs), since these terms have their own listing, with detailed descriptions, in section 4.14, in the chapter on sexual hygiene.

Appendix B

I also hope that this glossary will help the editors of standard dictionaries and interlingual dictionaries as they consider these terms and their meanings for possible inclusion in future editions of their reference works.

♥ ♥ ♥

-ad. A general suffix that means "a group of" (a specified number of things or people). The adjective form is *-adic* (e.g., *dyadic, triadic*). The number in the group is indicated by the first part of the word, from the Greek name for the number (because the suffix *-ad* is also of Greek origin). Thus, a "monad" is one of something, a single item, standing alone—a group of one, so to speak (a term not usually used in polyamory). A "dyad" is a group of two; and, in the context of polyamory, it means essentially a committed twosome, hence a somewhat narrower term than "couple" (see those terms herein). A "triad" in polyamory is a committed threesome, similar to the old French term *"ménage à trois"*, but there are subtle differences (so again, see those terms herein). Following this system of word formation, a committed foursome should be called a "tetrad", but in the actual poly community the term "quad" has come into general usage in English for this concept. A group of five committed people would be a "pentad", then a "hexad", "heptad", and so on, but in actuality groups this large tend to be loosely called a "clan", "tribe", "community", "family", etc.

affair. In mainstream culture, an ongoing sexual involvement by two people, at least one of whom is married or similarly committed to someone else. The underlying, unstated assumption is that such outside relationships are always in secret and in violation of the (explicit or tacit) vows of each spouse or primary partner to be

Appendix B

sexually exclusive, and are therefore a breach of trust, disrespectful, harmful. In polyamory, although not often used, the term "affair" could be applied to a secondary relationship carried on without the knowledge of one's primary partner(s), again in violation of explicit or tacit agreements. (See also "cheat".)

agreement. (Also called "relationship agreement".) An explicit understanding, written or unwritten, among primary partners (or possibly among others) spelling out the terms under which they agree to conduct their own relationship and any other intimate relationships. A relationship agreement typically spells out the safe sex practices that are to be used, the ways in which the partners are to communicate about secondary relationships, when and how one is to conduct secondary relationships, etc. The relationship agreement can also spell out financial arrangements or anything else agreed upon between or among the partners. Also see Chapter 5.

BDSM. An acronym for *bondage and discipline* (the first two letters), *dominance and submission* (the middle two letters), and *sadomasochism* (the last two letters). See each of those terms separately. Not related to polyamory; a person can enjoy BDSM relationships or polyamory or both or neither.

bi. A clipped form of "bisexual", used as an adjective or noun (plural in the noun sense: "bis"); ***bi-curious***: having no experience so far in sexual expression with someone of the same gender (if one identifies as heterosexual) or of the other gender (if homosexual), but interested in trying it.

biamory. (Pronounced "by-AM-ur-ee". Adjective form: *biamorous*, "by-AM-ur-us".) The personality orientation in which a person can be content in either a monamorous or polyamorous relationship.

bigamy. Marriage to two spouses simultaneously. (See *marriage*.)

bisexual. (Adjective or noun.) Referring to a person who enjoys sex with both men and women.

bondage and discipline. A form of sexual expression in which one person agrees to be physically restricted in some way (tied to the bed, hands tied together, blindfolded, etc.) while their partner or partners do sexually stimulating things to them. The participants always agree on a "safe word" which the one bound or restricted can utter to gain immediate release from their bondage; when cords and knots are used, they are typically arranged so that the person bound can pull them loose without help.

bottom. In gay sex, the man who is penetrated. (Also see *top*.)

cheat. In mainstream culture, to engage in any sexual activity outside one's marriage or comparable commitment. The underlying, unstated assumption is that married or committed partners have always vowed sexual exclusivity, explicitly or implicitly, so that any such outside relationship constitutes a violation of the vows, i.e., cheating. In polyamory, although not often used, the term would mean engaging in a sexual relationship outside one's marriage or commitment in violation of the provisions of one's explicit relationship agreement, or behaving in a secondary relationship contrary to one's relationship agreement, for example by not using condoms if the agreement requires them. (Also see *affair; relationship agreement*.)

clan. Loosely, any group of more than about four adults (with any children involved) who consider themselves to be a chosen family (whether or not living together), typically with polyamorous sexual involvement among some or all of the adults. Similar to *tribe*.

closet. The practice of keeping one's sexual orientation or lifestyle (such as homosexuality, polyamory, or BDSM) secret from general knowledge; ***closeted***: same as "in the closet"; ***come out of the closet***:

Appendix B

after a period of secrecy, let friends, family, associates, or anyone else know of one's homosexual, polyamorous, etc., lifestyle; ***in the closet***: maintaining secrecy about one's homosexual, polyamorous, etc., lifestyle; ***out of the closet***: allowing general knowledge about one's homosexual, polyamorous, etc., lifestyle. (Also see *out*.)

co-housing. A type of intentional community commonly found in urban and suburban areas, but which may also be rural, in which a group of people live in adjacent housing units and share varying degrees of work, social interaction, ownership of real estate, etc.

co-husband. A term that can be used by a man in a triad or larger polyamorous family in referring to another man (another husband) in the family. Many such families, however, use the simpler terms "husband", "wife", or "partner".

commitment. A firm mutual promise between primary partners to stay in a personal relationship and work together through difficulties diligently and in good faith unless or until it becomes apparent, in spite of diligent good-faith attempts at resolution, that there are problems so serious that they render it impractical or inadvisable to one or both or all partners to stay in the relationship.

community. A group of people or subset of the population with similar interests, philosophy, lifestyle, etc.; for example, the polyamory community or the lesbian community. ***Intentional community:*** a group of people living on a shared piece of land, with admission to the community subject to approval by existing members; usually also with some common philosophy, purpose, lifestyle, means of support, etc. Many but not all intentional communities include polyamory among some or all adult community members. There are wide differences in the degree of economic sharing, work sharing, the sharing of meals and personal living spaces, ownership of real estate, and other structural and behavioral details. Also see "co-housing" and "ecovillage".

Appendix B

compersion. (Pronunciation: "kum-PURR-zhun". Adjective: *compersive,* pronounced "kum-PURR-siv".) Empathetic feelings of joy and satisfaction when one's loving partner shares sex with someone else, or has a loving relationship with someone else. Sometimes thought of as the opposite of jealousy. An equivalent in the United Kingdom, New Zealand, and Australia is *frubble;* adjective, *frubbly.*

couple. Two people in a loving relationship or having some other interpersonal involvement. The term is variously used to refer to two people who are married or living together or simply physically present together at the moment, e.g. on a date. This distinguishes the term from *dyad,* which is used in a narrower sense to refer only to two people in a committed loving relationship, usually living together. (In other contexts, the word *couple* is also used to refer to two people with the briefest of connections, for example, two people dancing together.)

co-wife. A term that can be used by a woman in a triad or larger polyamorous family in referring to another woman (another wife) in the family. Many such families, however, use the simpler terms "husband" and "wife".

curious. Having no experience so far in some form of relationship or sexual expression, but interested in trying it. Used in hyphenated forms such as "bi-curious" or "poly-curious".

dom. A clipped form of "dominant" (noun), or "dominant person".

dominance. A preference, by the nature of one's personality, to be in an authoritative, superior position over one's sexual partner(s), giving orders, making decisions, etc. See also *dominant.*

dominant. As an adjective, referring to *dominance.* As a noun, a person who enjoys dominance in personal or sexual relationships. As a noun, often clipped to *dom;* **dominant/submissive** (abbreviated

Appendix B

"d/s" or "D/s"): referring to the type of relationship between a dominant person and a submissive person.

double penetration (often abbreviated "DP"). Simultaneous penetration of a woman's vagina and anus by two men's penises.

DP. Abbreviation of "double penetration".

d/s, D/s. Abbreviation of "dominant/submissive" (see under *dominant*).

dyad. (Adjective: *dyadic*.) A group of two mutually committed people in a loving relationship, usually living together. This makes the term *dyad* somewhat narrower than *couple*. The word *dyad* is also used more often when the context includes reference to committed groups of larger numbers as well, i.e., dyads, triads, quads, etc.

ecovillage. A type of intentional community that strives for ecological (environmental) responsibility and sustainability by minimizing their consumption of nonrenewable resources, using renewable resources sustainably, and living as self-sufficiently as they can with regard to food, water, and energy.

faithful. In mainstream culture, this term refers to a person who is sexually exclusive with their spouse or comparable committed partner. The unstated assumption is that every married or similarly committed person automatically vows sexual exclusivity, explicitly or implicitly, so that "faithful" equates to keeping that presumed promise of exclusivity. In polyamory, although the word is not often used, it would mean adhering to one's relationship agreement. (See also *cheat; relationship agreement*.)

family. A group of two or more adults who have chosen to be emotionally intimate, along with any children involved, usually but not always also living together and with the adults usually relating sexually in one or more combinations; ***chosen family:*** the people with whom someone chooses to live or have a close association, based on mutual

Appendix B

love or affection; ***family of origin:*** the family in which one was raised through childhood; ***extended family:*** the larger group of one's traditional relatives, including not only parents and children but also grandparents, uncles and aunts, cousins, etc.; ***nuclear family,*** husband, wife, and children, or (sometimes) a separated or widowed parent with child or children, not including grandparents, aunts, uncles, etc. The term could also apply to a gay or lesbian dyad and their children.

fetish. An object not usually associated with sex but used by a person for sexual stimulation; e.g., a feather duster, leather, candle wax, the underwear of the other gender, etc.; ***fetishism:*** the practice or enjoyment of using fetishes.

fluid-bonded. Referring to two or more people who share sex without condoms or other physical barriers, or who have mutual sexual partners who do so, so that there is a direct person-to-person-to-person linkage, allowing the microbes in bodily fluids to pass among the people involved. That is, two or more people are fluid-bonded if they exchange bodily fluids (especially vaginal fluids, semen, blood, urine, or rectal and fecal moisture—the means by which STDs are typically transmitted) directly or through one or more shared partners during sexual involvement.

FMF. (Acronym for "female-male-female".) Referring to a triad or other threesome consisting of two women and a man.

foursome. See *"-some"*.

friend with benefits. A friend with whom one shares sex. Such friends may or may not have an emotional connectedness in addition to the sexual involvement. This is a more formal and broadly acceptable term than the synonymous *fuck-buddy*.

frubble. An equivalent in the United Kingdom, New Zealand, and Australia for *compersion,* which see. Adjective: *frubbly.*

Appendix B

fuck-buddy. A more informal and sometimes socially disapproved synonym for *friend with benefits*.

gang-bang. A sexual encounter involving a number of men and one woman, all of the men sharing sex with the woman simultaneously or in sequence.

gay. (Adjective or noun.) A homosexual male. Sometimes used to include lesbians when gender is not relevant to the context, as in "gay rights", "gay marriage".

GLBT. Acronym for "gay, lesbian, bisexual, and transsexual" (same as "LGBT").

hermaphrodite. (Adjective: *hermaphroditic.*) A person born with the physical sexual characteristics of both male and female to one degree or another, typically also with gender-mixed hormones. Such persons are often surgically altered soon after birth to give them the more "normal" physical appearance of one or the other gender. A synonym of *hermaphroditic* is *intersexed*.

het, hetero. Clipped forms of *heterosexual*.

heterosexual. (Adjective or noun.) Referring to a person who enjoys sex only with persons of the other gender. Often clipped as *het* or *hetero*.

hexad. An intimate, committed group of six adults.

homosexual. (Adjective or noun.) Referring to a person who enjoys sex only with persons of his or her own gender.

hot seat. The situation in which one member of a triad or larger primary group is confronted (lovingly and compassionately) on an issue by two or more primary partners, so that the partner being confronted cannot fall back on asserting "you have your opinion and I have mine," as in a dyad, but is obliged to take the remarks of the other partners seriously and engage in introspection to understand their position and perhaps undergo personal change and growth; for

Appendix B

example, "The hot seat phenomenon is unique to triads and larger primary groups;" "All four of us in the quad found ourselves in the hot seat at different times."

IC. Acronym for "intentional community" (see under "community").

incubation period. The time between when a microbe first infects a body with a disease and when symptoms of disease first appear or the disease can be detected by medical tests. Even during the incubation period when the infection is not detectable, the disease can usually already be passed on to other persons; that is, the newly infected person is contagious.

intentional community. See under "community".

intersexed. Referring to a person born with the physical sexual characteristics of both male and female to one degree or another; hermaphroditic.

intimate. Closely sharing with another person. People are *physically intimate* if they are sexually involved with each other. They are *emotionally intimate* if they express their own feelings and want to know about the other's feelings deeply and thoroughly.

jealous. (Noun: *jealousy*.) Feeling resentment, anger, and fear when one's loving partner shares sexually with someone else, or has a loving relationship with someone else. Jealous feelings can also occur when someone only suspects or contemplates the possibility that their loving partner may be or might become physically or emotionally intimate with someone else. Also see *compersion*.

kink. (Adjective: *kinky*.) A loose term referring to any style of sexual expression (either heterosexual or homosexual) that involves an additional component in addition to what mainstream culture considers "normal"; e.g., fetishism, or BDSM.

LDR. Acronym for "long-distance relationship" (see under "relationship").

Appendix B

LGBT. Acronym for "lesbian, gay, bisexual, and transgendered" (same as "GLBT").

lesbian. (Adjective or noun.) A homosexual woman.

lifestyle. Any manner in which one chooses to conduct one's life. Among swingers, "the lifestyle" is used as a code phrase synonymous with "swinging"; for example, "We have been in the lifestyle for five years;" "Do you enjoy lifestyle parties?"

line marriage. See under *marriage*.

LM. Acronym for "Loving More", a polyamory organization.

mainstream. (Adjective or noun.) Referring to the dominant, majority culture of a region. In the western hemisphere and Europe, this refers to the traditional culture that assumes (among other things) that all intimate interpersonal relationships must be heterosexual, dyadic, and sexually exclusive.

marriage. Registration of a personal partnership with the government, thereby bestowing certain legal rights to the partners and their offspring, or the state of having registered one's partnership with the government (with no revocation). Although religious clergy as well as certain government officials commonly conduct "marriage" ceremonies, it is not a legally valid marriage unless the local government's laws recognize it as such. ***Group marriage:*** a term coined around the middle of the 20th century to describe a marriage-like committed group of more than two partners (not legally recognized as a marriage)—a broader term that includes a triad, quad, clan, etc. ***Line marriage:*** a type of marriage or committed group envisioned in the 1960s and 1970s by the science fiction author Robert H. Heinlein, in which younger adults occasionally join a group marriage, as elderly partners die off, thus maintaining an approximately stable number of partners indefinitely, potentially over centuries. Some modern polyamorous families have adopted

Appendix B

the line marriage concept, including the term. ***Open marriage:*** essentially the same as *open relationship,* when the couple in question is married (see *open relationship,* under *relationship*).

masochism. Sexual arousal by receiving pain and discomfort from another person. (Also see *sadism* and *sadomasochism.*)

masochist. One who enjoys *masochism.*

master. An extremely dominant person, especially but not always a man. (The female equivalent is "mistress".) A master typically enjoys controlling not only his partner's sexual activities, but most or all other aspects of his partner's life as well, such as who the other person forms friendships with, who else they share sex with, what they do and say, etc. The other person in such a relationship is known as a "slave".

ménage à trois. An old French term referring to a sexual threesome; it literally means "group of three". Among polyamorous people, the term *triad* more often than not refers to a threesome living together, while a *ménage à trois* may or may not live together, and may be a casual sexual threesome. Polyamorous people usually refer to a more casual three-person sexual encounter as a *threesome.*

MFM. (Acronym for "male-female-male".) Referring to a triad or other threesome consisting of two men and a woman.

mistress. The female equivalent of a *master.*

monamory. (Pronunciation: "mon-AM-ur-ee". Adjective: *monamorous.* The clipped form "mono" is sometimes used to mean "monamorous".) The practice or theory of being sexually intimate with only one person at a time (sexually exclusive); contrasted to *polyamory.* (Also see *monogamy, polyamory,* and *biamory.*)

mono. A clipped form of *monamorous* or *monogamous.*

monogamy. (Adjective: *monogamous.* The clipped form *mono* is sometimes used for either *monogamy* and *monogamous,* as well as

Appendix B

monamory.) (1) The practice or legal requirement that a person may have only one (legal) spouse at a time (see *marriage*); (2) sometimes used with the same meaning as *monamory*. **Serial monogamy:** A somewhat humorous term referring to the prevalent phenomenon whereby a person marries, divorces, remarries, sometimes divorces and remarries further, thus having a series of mates but (officially) never more than one at a time.

munch. (Noun.) A gathering of a local polyamory group (or other group) at a restaurant for socializing over dinner.

new relationship energy (abbreviated "NRE"). The intense mutual feelings of love, excitement, and fascination among two or more people when their emotionally and/or sexually intimate relationship is relatively new.

NRE. Acronym for *new relationship energy*.

number tendency. A person's fundamental tendency (whether innate, like sexual orientation, or conditioned in childhood or later) to want either multiple loving relationships (polyamory) or only one at a time (monamory), or to be content with either arrangement; that is, the inclination to be either polyamorous, monamorous, or biamorous.

one-night stand. A sexual encounter with a person that occurs only once and is not repeated.

open. (1) In polyamory, not hiding information about one's other sexually intimate relationships, but fully sharing information about one's feelings and intimate involvements at least with one's primary partner(s), and others if appropriate; (2) not secretive with the general public about one's sexual and/or emotional lifestyle (although the personal identities of one's sexual partners may be kept confidential to protect the other person's privacy); casually acknowledging or mentioning that one is polyamorous, homosexual, etc., when that is relevant in conversation; "out of the closet".

orientation. A natural, inborn (not cultural or chosen) inclination to be attracted to one or another type of sexual relationship; ***sexual orientation***: the innate inclination to be attracted sexually either to the other gender or one's own gender or both (i.e., to be either heterosexual, homosexual, or bisexual). The tendency to want either polyamory or monamory, or to be content with either (what I refer to as "number tendency") may be an orientation, at least for some people.

OSO. Acronym for "other significant other". (See *significant other.*)

out. Used as an adjective: short for "out of the closet" (see "closet"). Used as a transitive verb: to disclose the sexual lifestyle of someone else against that person's wishes (involuntarily force that person "out of the closet"); for example, "After they broke up, Bob outed his former partner Tom to Tom's employer."

partner. (1) A person with whom one has a primary commitment, based on deep mutual love; (2) any person with whom one has an intimate involvement of some sort, including ongoing but less intense loving and sexual relationships or a once-only sexual involvement just for the enjoyment of the sex with little or no emotional connectedness. ***Domestic partner:*** a person with whom one lives in an emotionally and sexually intimate relationship (therefore excluding roommates). ***Life partner:*** a person with whom one has a primary commitment with the goal or intention that the partnership will endure as long as both or all partners are living. ***Primary partner:*** the person, or one of the people, with whom one has the deepest, most emotionally intimate relationship and the strongest commitment (in a triad or larger, sex may or may not be shared between two specific primary partners, depending on sexual orientation). ***Secondary partner:*** a person with whom one has an emotional and/or sexual involvement that is less intense, deep, or committed than a primary relationship,

Appendix B

so that, in the event of conflict, interactions with the secondary partner may yield to the higher priority of the primary relationship;. ***Tertiary partner*** (infrequently used term): a person with whom one has some degree of connection, usually including sex, but even less emotional attachment than with a secondary partner; a *tertiary partner* may be similar to a *friend with benefits* or *fuck-buddy*.

pentad. An intimate, committed group of five adults.

poly. (Adjective or noun.) A clipped form of *polyamory* or *polyamorous*. Used as a noun, it can also mean "polyamorous person"; in the latter sense, the plural form is "polys"; ***poly-curious:*** having no experience so far in polyamory but interested in trying it; ***poly/mono:*** referring to a dyadic relationship in which, by agreement, one partner is polyamorous, the other monamorous.

polyamory. (In countries other than the United States, usually spelled "polyamoury". Pronounced "pah-lee-AM-ur-ee". Adjective: *polyamorous* or *polyamourous,* pronounced "pah-lee-AM-ur-us". The clipped form "poly" ("PAH-lee") is often used to mean "polyamory", "polyamorous", or "polyamorous person". In the latter sense, the plural form "polys" is used. Also see *poly* for combined forms. The word was reportedly coined by Morning Glory Zell and first appeared publicly in an article she wrote and published in the periodical *The Green Egg* in 1990. Polyamory is the practice or theory of having emotionally intimate relationships with more than one person simultaneously, with sex as a permissible expression of the caring feelings, openly and honestly keeping one's primary partners (or dating partners) informed of the existence of other intimate involvements. Polyamory and swinging are somewhat overlapping concepts, but as generally used the terms are distinguished in that polyamory stresses the *emotional* connectedness of a person with multiple other persons (while sexual involvement is usually but not always also present or at least accepted as an option), while swinging stresses the *sexual* aspect of a person's relationships with multiple partners, typically primarily for the enjoyment of sex and of sexual variety. There are also other similarities and differences between polyamory and swinging that result from those first-level comparisons. The major similarity is openly sharing with one's primary partner the fact that one has other sexual involvements, and acceptance that one's primary partner is likewise involved. Both polyamory and swinging stress the importance of respecting other people and their preferences, limitations, etc. (e.g. accepting "no" without pressuring another person). Some prominent differences: (a) polyamorists as a group are more inclined to be out of the closet or are closeted only from concern for personal reprisals, e.g. from employers or family, while swingers have always tended to be more secretive and show little inclination toward political activism to get swinging accepted by the mainstream as a social option; (b) polyamorists show more variety of personal living arrangements, with many triads, quads, and the like, and have a much higher percentage of gays, lesbians, and bisexuals, whereas swingers are more predominantly heterosexual couples, and swinging organizations often look askance at single men and gay men; committed triads and quads are rare among swingers; (c) although there are no good data on this, swingers on average seem to be politically and religiously more conservative, while polyamorists typically are politically more progressive, and larger numbers of polyamorists are followers of alternative spiritual communities such as Paganism or Wicca, or are members of tolerant, accepting traditional spiritual communities such as Unitarian Universalism or Reform Judaism.

polyandry. (Adjective: *polyandrous*.) Marriage by a woman to two or more men simultaneously. (See *marriage*.)

Appendix B

polyfi. Clipped form of "polyfidelity" or "polyfidelitous".

polyfidelity. (Pronunciation: "pah-lee-fih-DEL-ih-tee". Adjective: *polyfidelitous,* "pah-lee-fih-DEL-ih-tous". Sometimes clipped to "polyfi" for both the noun and adjective.) Sexual exclusivity within a committed group or family of more than two adults. Thus, persons in a group practicing polyfidelity may be sexually intimate with anyone else within the group but promise never to share sex with anyone outside the group.

polygamy. (Adjective: *polygamous*.) Marriage by a person to two or more people simultaneously, without regard to gender. Thus, *polygamy* includes both polyandry and polygyny. (See *marriage*.)

polygyny. (Adjective: *polygynous*.) Marriage by a man to two or more women simultaneously. (See *marriage*.)

polyphobe. A polyphobic person.

polyphobia. (Adjective: *polyphobic*.) Bigoted disapproval of polyamory and polyamorous people.

polysexuality. Sexual activity with three or more people participating.

postop. A clipped form of *postoperative.*

postoperative. Referring to a transsexual who has received surgery to bring their physical characteristics more closely in line with their self-identified gender. Sometimes clipped to *postop*.

preop. A clipped form of *preoperative.*

preoperative. Referring to a transsexual who has not received surgery to bring their physical characteristics more closely in line with their self-identified gender. Sometimes clipped to *preop*.

primary. (Adjective or noun.) Referring to a relationship or partner with whom one has the greatest degree of love, emotional intimacy, and commitment; contrasted to *secondary*. Used as a noun, it is equivalent to "primary partner". Some polyamorists prefer not to use the terms "primary" and "secondary", feeling that they do not wish to rank their partners or relationships by importance or priority. Others are comfortable with these terms, because one or more of their relationships do have greater depth and importance for them, and therefore take priority in their lives. Typically, for someone who is married or comparably committed, their spouse or cohabiting partner(s) are primary, and outside intimate relationships are secondary (typically involving dates rather than living together). A single person with several dating relationships may or may not consider one relationship to be primary.

quad. An intimate, committed group of four adults.

queer. (Adjective or noun.) Originally a derogatory term for a homosexual, the gay and lesbian communities have reclaimed the word and use it themselves to describe themselves and their community. The word is also sometimes expanded to include transgendered persons and those who enjoy various kinks.

recreational sex. Enjoyment of sex with numerous partners simply for the fun of the sex, commonly with little or no emotional connection between partners. This is a large component of swinging, but those who identify themselves as swingers often assert that swinging is a broader phenomenon, often including deep friendships and warm emotional relationships among participants—which moves into the overlap area between swinging and polyamory. (Also see *swinging*.)

relationship. An ongoing emotional and/or sexual involvement between two or more people. **Barter relationship:** my term for a relationship based on an explicit or tacit agreement whereby one person agrees to do what the other wants if the other will do what the first person wants—a basically self-centered attitude by both partners. **Long-distance relationship** (abbreviated "LDR"): one

Appendix B

in which the persons involved are separated geographically to the extent that meeting in person is time-consuming and expensive. ***Open relationship:*** a marriage or other dyadic relationship in which the partners agree to allow sexual involvement with others, without secrecy; this term encompasses both swinging and polyamory. ***Primary relationship:*** a relationship that is given first ranking and priority in one's life because it entails the greatest depth of love, commitment, and daily interactions. ***Secondary relationship:*** a relationship that is less central in one's life than a primary relationship, because of lesser love, commitment, and daily interactions. Typically a primary relationship entails living together, and a secondary relationship involves living separately and dating. Also see the commentary under *primary*.

sadism. Sexual arousal by inflicting pain and discomfort on another person. (Also see *masochism* and *sadomasochism*.)

sadist. One who enjoys *sadism*.

sadomasochism. A form of sexual expression in which one person (the sadist) is sexually aroused by inflicting pain and discomfort of one sort or another on another person, while the other person (the masochist) is aroused by receiving pain and discomfort. (Adjective: *sadomasochistic*.)

safe word. In BDSM, a word which the submissive (physically bound) person can utter when they wish to stop the sexual play and have the other person(s) immediately untie the cords etc. that restrict them. The other sexual partner is then obligated by honor to release the bound person.

scene. In BDSM, a (usually) prearranged sexual session that involves role-playing and acting out a simple or involved dramatic situation. For example, one partner might play the role of a misbehaving child in need of punishment while the other person acts as parent or teacher, administering spanking or other punishment, which is sexually arousing; or one partner might play the role of a person in need of rescuing, while the other person is the rescuer; doctor and patient; etc.

secondary. (Adjective or noun.) Referring to a partner or relationship that is less central or important in one's life than another partner or relationship (which is "primary"). Used as a noun, it is equivalent to "secondary partner". While secondary relationships are also treated with respect and ethical behavior, activities with a secondary may occasionally need to yield to scheduling conflicts or conflicting needs or desires within the primary relationship. In some cases, if a person's primary partner is uncomfortable even with the existence of the secondary relationship, that person may be honor-bound to terminate the secondary relationship for the sake of honesty within the primary relationship and to preserve the primary relationship. Also see *primary, relationship,* and *special friend.*

sexually transmitted disease. (Often abbreviated "STD".) Any infectious disease that can be transmitted by one or another form of sexual expression. Many STDs can also be transmitted in nonsexual ways.

slave. An extremely submissive person, who voluntarily relinquishes assertiveness and self-choice not just in the sexual realm but also in most other aspects of life to another person, whom they consider to be their *master* or *mistress*.

slut. (Adjective: *slutty.*) Originally a derogatory term for a woman who is sexually active with various partners; the term has been reclaimed by many, on the basis that sex is a positive, joyous experience for both genders, and having multiple partners is not ethically reprehensible. There is no equivalent derogatory term in English for promiscuous men, except for the weaker term "womanizer" or "Don Juan" (after

Appendix B

the opera character), since mainstream culture has considered promiscuity among men to be at least tacitly admirable and so has applied approving terms to such men (e.g., "stud").

significant other. A term used both in the poly community and elsewhere to refer to a person with whom one has an emotionally and/or sexually close relationship, either on the level of dating or cohabitation; often abbreviated *SO*. ***Other significant other:*** in polyamory, synonymous with *secondary partner;* often abbreviated *OSO*.

SO. Acronym for *significant other*.

-some. A general suffix meaning "a group of" (a number indicated by the beginning of the word), thus an Anglo-Saxon equivalent of "-ad"; for example, "twosome", "threesome", "foursome". In polyamory, "-some" terms do not indicate any degree of closeness or commitment, so a threesome might be a casual get-together (sexual or not) of three friends, or a committed triad, or anything between.

special friend. A substitute term for "secondary partner" useful when speaking to children in a poly household who are too young to understand romance or sex. For example, "Mom is on the phone with her special friend Bob." The term might also be useful in other contexts.

STD. Acronym for *sexually transmitted disease*.

STI. Acronym for *sexually transmitted infection,* a term equivalent to "STD".

straight. Originally (in the sexual context) meaning "heterosexual", and still usually used in that sense; the term is also sometimes used to refer to someone not in another category, e.g., not kinky, not a drug user, etc.

sub. A clipped form of "submissive".

submissive. (Adjective or noun.) Referring to a person who prefers to yield to another (a "dominant" person) in making choices and decisions in the sexual realm or otherwise. (Often clipped to "sub". Also see *dominant.*)

swinger. A person who enjoys swinging.

swinging. A form of sexually open behavior in which a person enjoys a variety of sexual partners, usually in a social setting, e.g. club sex parties or private gatherings of friends. There is some overlap between swinging and polyamory, although there are major differences beyond the common factor of open sexuality, such that the two communities, polyamory and swinging, are mostly distinct. Also see *polyamory* and *recreational sex.*

switch. In BDSM, a person who enjoys sometimes playing a dominant role in sex, sometimes a submissive role.

tertiary. A term infrequently but occasionally used to refer to a sexual partner with whom there is an even more tenuous, shallow emotional involvement than is suggested by the term "secondary". See also *tertiary partner* under *partner.*

tetrad. In the general system of nomenclature for groups (see *–ad*), a committed loving group of four; however, in practice, a group of four is usually called a *quad.*

they. (Derived forms *them, their, theirs,* as in the plural sense, but with the new reflexive form *themself.* Used with the plural verb form. The singular use of this pronoun, and the plural verb form, follows the example of the pronoun "you", originally plural only, then extended to singular usage with the reflexive pronoun "yourself" but retaining the plural verb.) When used in a singular sense, equivalent to "he or she, as the case may be"; for example, "A polyamorous person's primary partner is entitled to complete and honest answers when they ask for information.")

Appendix B

threesome. See "*-some*".

top. In gay sex, the man who penetrates. (Also see *bottom*.)

tranny. A clipped form of "transsexual".

transgendered. Transsexual (adjective).

transsexual. (Adjective or noun.) Referring to a person who feels that the gender identity of their personality does not match their physical characteristics (e.g., a person who "feels" male in a body with breasts and vagina; a person who "feels" female in a body with penis and facial hair); also referring to the concerns, issues, etc., of transsexual persons. Many transsexuals obtain surgery and hormone therapy to allow their physical characteristics to match their self-identified gender to the extent possible; hence a transsexual may be either *preoperative* or *postoperative* (or *preop* or *postop*). Being transsexual is not a sexual orientation, since "orientation" refers to how one is attracted sexually to other people, while transsexuality refers to how one identifies one's own gender. ("Transsexual" is sometimes colloquially clipped to "tranny".)

triad. An intimate, committed group of three adults. Also see *ménage à trois*.

triangle. A triad or other threesome in which all three twosome combinations are sexual with each other (not necessarily at the same time).

tribe. A loosely defined term for a somewhat large community of people who feel that they share values, emotional connectedness, worldviews, etc., and often with sexual sharing among various members. A tribe commonly lives in geographical proximity, but not always. Similar to *clan*.

twosome. A sexual encounter or sharing involving two people (who may have any degree of emotional bonding, or none).

V. (Also called a "vee".) A triad or a more casual threesome in which two of the three people are not sexually involved with each other, but both are sexual with the same third person (that is, person A with B, B with C, but not A with C); ***emotional V (or vee):*** a triad or more casual threesome in which there is little or no emotional connectedness between two of the people.

vanilla. Used as an adjective, usually in the BDSM community, to refer to sexual activity that does not include any form of kink; or to a person who does not enjoy any form of kink.

vee. Same as "V".

W. A pentad or a more casual fivesome in which person A is sexually intimate with B, B with C, C with D, and D with E, but no other combinations share sex.

WPA. Acronym for the World Polyamory Association.

Y. A quad or more casual foursome in which A is sexually intimate with B, C, and D, but there is no direct sexual involvement among B, C, and D.

Z. A quad or more casual foursome in which A is sexually intimate with B, B with C, and C with D, with no direct sexual involvement in other pairings.

~ Appendix C ~

Quick Quirk Quotient Questionnaire

See sections 1.05 and 9.07 for a discussion of this questionnaire and the factors behind it.

This questionnaire is designed for those who have recently met, or already have a relationship on the secondary or friendship level, and who are considering the wisdom of forming a primary partnership. Certainly those who are already primary partners can also benefit from taking this questionnaire. Doing so may help you identify some areas where you would benefit by discussing the question and then agreeing on how you and your primary partner(s) can live with the differences.

This questionnaire is certainly not an exhaustive list of all the concerns or questions that two or more people should think about when they are considering whether to form a primary partnership.

The questionnaire is just as relevant for single persons seeking one primary partner as for those hoping to form a triad or larger primary group.

Each question stands alone, and so there is no meaning in adding up your points to all the questions. There are no "right", "wrong", or "better" answers. The point here is for you and potential new partners to learn about each other and think about some factors that could loom important in your lives, especially if you decide to live together. So, after everyone has finished, compare your answer to each question to how each other person answered that question. The closer you and the other person(s) are to the same rating on that question, the more compatible you are on that item.

Appendix C

If you both or all of you score similarly on most of the questions, you're fortunate! You could expect a relatively easier time being primary partners.

If there are significant discrepancies in your scores to many questions, this doesn't mean that you can't be successful as primaries, but you can expect more substantial issues between you if you live together, so you may want to think about whether you'd be better off being secondary partners or nonsexual friends.

Keep in mind, though, that in many cases polyamory helps primaries live more comfortably with substantial differences of these sorts. For example, suppose your favorite recreation is bicycling or skiing but your primary would rather read a book or crochet; or your ideal vacation is to loll on a warm beach sipping piñas coladas, while your partner would rather do a hut-to-hut snowshoeing trek. This sort of difference can be a major bone of contention for monamorous partners who have no one else close in their lives. But for you, being poly, you can find a secondary who enjoys the same kinds of activities that you do, while your primary follows their preferences with a secondary of their own. You then come back from your times with your secondary and tell your primary how invigorating the snowshoe trek was or how relaxing that beach was. Hopefully, of course, you and your primary(-ies) also have plenty of things on which you resonate in your lives, to provide the "glue" for your relationship.

There are some factors, of course, where sharing with a secondary will not help get beyond a difference between primaries. For example, if you don't smoke and you detest the odor of tobacco smoke but your partner or a potential new partner strongly wants to be able to smoke in the home, this is obviously a huge obstacle to a successful cohabiting partnership. The same is true if you like loud rock music, or bagpipes, or opera, or Bulgarian women's choruses, but the other person can't stand your preferred musical styles.

Appendix C

There is no particular rank of importance to these questions, since different factors will hold varying importance to different people.

After you and each of your partners or potential new partners have completed the questionnaire, sit down to compare your answers, item by item. When the various answers to that item are the same or close, great. When you find differences of several points in your answers to a particular item, you and your partner(s) or potential partner(s) may want to discuss that item to decide whether you can comfortably live with your divergent feelings, or whether you can find flexibility to shift closer together or compromise, or whether the differences of attitudes are great enough, and your positions firm enough, that it would not be wise to try to form a primary partnership.

If you decide to go ahead with forming a primary partnership even though you've come upon some substantial differences in your answers to this questionnaire, you might want to consider including your resolution as to how you will deal with each of these items, after you've discussed each of them together, in your relationship agreement (see Chapter 5).

Photocopy these pages, one copy for each person who will be taking the questionnaire. Alternatively, each person can mark their answers on a blank piece of paper. Mark each question on a scale from 0 to 10, where:

0 = "I couldn't stand to have this in my life or live life this way;"
From 1 to 4 = degrees of "I don't like this, but I could tolerate it;"
5 = "I don't care one way or the other—whatever;"
From 6 to 9 = "I like this, but I could do without it if I had to;" and
10 = "This is very important or essential in my life."

Do this separately, not comparing answers until each of you has finished.

♥ ♥ ♥

Appendix C

_____ 1. Would you like to know lots of details about your primary's secondary partners and your primary's activities with their secondaries (in contrast to knowing only a few basic facts, such as a secondary's identity)?

_____ 2. Is it important to you to know your primary's secondary's primary?

_____ 3. Are you comfortable having your primary partner stay overnight with a secondary?

_____ 4. Are you comfortable having your primary take a multi-day trip with a secondary?

_____ 5. Are you comfortable seeing your primary show affection with a secondary in your presence (or hearing them on the phone etc.)?

_____ 6. Do you enjoy sex involving yourself, your primary, and one or more others (polysexuality)?

_____ 7. Are you comfortable being open (out of the closet) about your polyamorous lifestyle or orientation?

_____ 8. Do you like to keep your living quarters clean and tidy, putting everything away as soon as you're done with it, washing the dishes or loading the dishwasher after every meal, being sure dirty clothes make it immediately into the hamper?

Appendix C

_____ 9. Is it important to you to follow certain dietary customs, such as keeping kosher or following an organic, vegetarian, vegan, or carnivorous diet?

_____ 10. Is it important to you to have a smoke-free environment at home?

_____ 11. Is it important to you to have a cat?

_____ 12. Is it important to you to have a dog?

_____ 13. When there are no outside influences on your sleep times, such as work schedules, do you tend to stay up till the wee hours, then sleep till mid morning or noon?

_____ 14. Do you like to watch a lot of TV during your free time?

_____ 15. Do you like to have music (of whatever sort) playing most of the time at home or in the car?

_____ 16. When you have music playing at home or in the car, is it important to you that it be one of your preferred styles?

_____ 17. Do you prefer noncommercial or listener-sponsored radio or TV stations over those that carry commercials?

_____ 18. Do you enjoy socializing with lots of people (i.e., are you an extrovert)?

_____ 19. Is it important to you to be active in a particular organized religion, or to observe the rituals and holidays of a particular spiritual or religious practice?

Appendix C

_____ 20. Is it important to you to pursue personal spiritual growth and development (whether or not as part of an organized religion)?

_____ 21. Is it important to you to make a minimal "footprint" on the environment by your life, that is, permaculture, local economy, intentional community, recycling, reducing or minimizing consumption of nonrenewable resources, minimizing the release of carbon dioxide into the atmosphere, etc.?

_____ 22. Is it important to you to do what you can to earn more money and increase your material standard of living?

_____ 23. Do you prefer to live in a densely populated, urban area (in contrast to rural or small-town environments)?

_____ 24. Do you prefer to live in a warm climate (in contrast to temperate or cold)?

_____ 25. Do you prefer to take vacations that are physically active (in contrast to cruises, lying on the beach, etc.)?

_____ 26. Do you prefer to take vacations to exotic or foreign places (in contrast to going only to one or two familiar places close to home, or staying home during vacations)?

_____ 27. Is it important to you for everything in your life to be just the way you want it, with everything done just the way you want it done (in contrast to "going with the flow" and letting others often decide things even when the decisions affect you)?

Appendix C

_____ 28. Do you like your home to be cool (sweater temperature) during the winter (in contrast to heating your home so that you are comfortable naked or in light clothing even during the winter)?

_____ 29. Are you comfortable with nudity at home?

_____ 30. Are you comfortable leaving the door open when the bathroom is in use?

_____ 31. Do you prefer to have the toilet paper come off the front of the roll, rather than the back side by the wall?

_____ 32. Do you like to pool all finances of the primary family, taking funds as needed for personal as well as shared expenses (in contrast to maintaining a joint account or "pot" in addition to one personal account for each partner, with each partner contributing to the joint account according to an agreed formula)?

_____ 33. If you have one or more minor children at home, and if you merge your household with one or more additional adults (who may or may not have children of their own), do you prefer for all adults to assume the role of parent equally for all children (in contrast to having the "original" parents retain the parental role for their own children alone, having a sort of buddy or mentor relationship with the other children in the household)?

~ *Index* ~

accidental exposure 4.02
acquaintanceship 6.08
activism, political 8.11
affairs
    general 3.01
    coming clean 3.03
    consequences 1.01
    motivation 1.01
agent, legal 10.03
agreement
    consensus 9.03
    relationship 5.01
    reluctant 7.12
AIDS 4.14
Alessandra, Tony 6.06
alphabet soup 2.12
alternate channels of communication 8.11
anal sex 4.02, 4.06
anger 7.07
approval of secondary 5.04
asking about health 4.03
attitudes 6.01, 6.13
attorney-in-fact 10.03
bacterial vaginosis 4.14
barter relationship 6.06, 7.05
bed arrangements 5.04, 9.03
beliefs 8.13
betrayal, causes of 1.01
bigotry
    general 8.13
    by government 10.07
biological parents 9.06

Index

bisexuals, suited to polyamory 1.04
black-and-white thinking 8.13
body piercing 4.01
breast-feeding 4.01, 4.02
Buddha 3.01
burnout 9.01
cerebrum 7.04
channels of communication, alternate 8.11
cheating in polyamory 6.13
childbirth 4.01, 4.02
childcare (in multi-adult families) 9.03
children
    acting on behalf 10.06
    biological parentage 10.06
    blossoming in multi-adult families 9.03
    care in multi-adult families 9.03
    child support 10.06
    custody 10.06, 10.09
    guardianship 10.04, 10.06
    hiding things from 6.11
    how they resolve conflicts 6.11
    in dyads 8.08
    in triads or larger 6.11, 9.06
    informing 5.04, 6.11, 8.08
    multiple parents 9.03
    of single parents 8.08
    parents end relationship 7.16, 9.12
    upon your death 10.04
chlamydia 4.14
choice or orientation 1.04
chores (multi-adult families) 9.03
clans 2.05, 9.05
clap, the 4.14
closet, the
    how 8.05
    not outing 3.08
    whether 8.04

Index

codicils ... 10.04
combinations, sexual ... 2.12
commitment ceremonies ... 10.11
communication
    general ... 6.01
    about secondaries ... 6.09
    beyond the basics ... 6.08
    channels ... 8.11
    childhood ... 6.08, 6.10
    don't ask, don't tell ... 6.07
    exponential ... 8.11
    feelings about secondary ... 6.09
    foundation of ... 6.06
    getting acquainted ... 6.08
    getting stuck ... 6.08
    hypothetical secondary ... 6.09
    Internet ... 8.11
    levels with primary ... 6.07
    new secondary ... 6.09
    probing psyches ... 6.08
    report/rapport ... 6.02
    sharing about self ... 6.08
    styles ... 6.02
    with secondary ... 6.10
communities ... 2.05, 2.07, 9.05
compersion ... 6.13
complexity in relationships ... 1.01, 9.02
compromise ... 6.13
condoms
    among primaries ... 7.07, 4.13
    breaking, slipping ... 4.04
    easier placement ... 4.12
    exceptions ... 5.04
    fluid-bonded ... 4.11
    starting after fluid-bonded ... 4.08
    using ... 4.02, 4.04, 4.06
confidentialities ... 3.08

Index

conscience, clearing 7.07
consensus 9.03
counseling 3.04, 7.14
couples dating others 2.03
crabs 4.14
custody 10.06, 10.09
dates, without primary 5.04
day-to-day life 8.01
defamation 10.10
deltas 2.12
demonstrations 8.11
dependents, minor or incompetent 10.04
digital stimulation 5.04
dildos 4.07
dilemmas 3.01, 3.07
discrimination 10.07
discussions 9.03
diseases
    heritable 9.06
    list of 4.14
    sexually transmitted 4.01
DNA testing 9.06
dom-sub games 6.13
don't ask, don't tell 6.07
dynamics
    general 2.04
    sexual, in foursomes 6.12
either-or thinking 8.13
emotional reactions 7.04
empathy 6.06, 6.13
ethics 3.01
everyday life 8.01
exceptions to condom use 5.04
executor of will 10.04
exposure to STDs 4.02
experiment 1.06

Index

expression of interest
- received by committed person ... 1.09
- to someone else ... 1.08

extrovert, introvert ... 1.04

families
- discussions ... 9.03
- meetings ... 9.10
- multi-adult ... 9.01

fear ... 7.05
fight or flight ... 7.04
fillers in speaking ... 8.12

finances
- general ... 5.04
- triads and larger ... 9.08

fingers etc. for sexual pleasure ... 4.12
fivesomes ... 9.05
flaws, personality ... 6.01, 6.08, 9.11
flexibility ... 6.13, 8.02
fluid-bonding ... (see "condoms")
foot-dragging ... 7.12
foursomes (sexual dynamics) ... 6.12
Franklin, Benjamin ... 8.05
frubble ... 6.13
genital warts ... 4.14
getting acquainted ... 6.08
getting stuck ... 6.08

Golden Rule
- general ... 3.01
- modifying ... 6.06

gonorrhea ... 4.14
goose and gander ... 2.08

groups
- global ... 8.09
- local ... 8.09
- starting ... 8.10

growing edges ... 6.01, 6.08, 9.11
guardianship ... 10.02, 10.04, 10.06

357

Index

guilt	7.10
hassles	10.07
health, asking about	4.03
hepatitis	4.14
heptads	2.05
herd thinking	10.07
herpes	4.14
hesitant agreement	7.12
hexads	2.05
HIV	4.14
hobbies	9.09
home	
buying	10.05
maintenance (multi-adult families)	9.03
homosexuals, suited to polyamory	1.04
hot buttons	7.04
hot seat	9.11
HPV	4.14
human papilloma virus	4.14
hygiene, sexual	4.01
hypothetical secondary	6.09
incompetent dependents	10.04
incubation period	4.10
indoctrination	8.13
inexperience	1.06
infection	4.01
infidelity	
one's own	7.07
partner confesses	7.09, 7.10
information	
for children	5.04
how much to share	5.04
withholding from primary	3.04, 5.04
informing dates, by single	2.02
inheritance	10.04
integrity	3.04
intentional communities	2.07, 9.05

Index

intestate	10.04
introvert, extrovert	1.04
issues	
attitudes	7.02
general	7.01
heal old stuff first	7.03
qualities for resolving	7.02
time and place	7.02
jealousy	1.09, 6.13, 7.05
karma	3.01
knowing oneself	6.01
leader role	9.05
leaving	9.12
legalities	10.01
libel	10.10
lice, pubic	4.14
limbic brain	7.04
living arrangements	9.07
living wills	10.02
majority, minority	9.03, 9.11
marriage	1.03, 10.11
massage	4.12, 8.10
meetings, family	9.10
men, single	1.02
menstruation	4.02, 4.04
mono-poly	2.08
moratoriums	
early	6.04
general	1.06
later	7.13
mortgages	10.05
multi-adult families	9.01
neighbors, meeting	8.05
networking	8.09
new relationship energy	6.04
Newton, Isaac	3.01
NGU	4.14

Index

nongonococcal urethritis	4.14
norms of society	5.01
NRE	6.04
one-sided open relationship	2.08
open-house party	8.05
openness and honesty	
conflicting values	3.04
general	1.01, 3.01, 6.07
oral sex	4.02, 4.05
ordinary life	8.01
organizing a local group	8.10
orientation or choice	1.04
out (of the closet)	8.03, 8.04, 8.05
outing	3.10
overnight with secondary	5.04
pacing oneself	9.01
pads, waterproof	4.04
parentage	
biological	9.06
testing	10.06
parents	
biological	9.06
dyads	8.08
single	8.08
triads and larger	9.06
partners	
finding	1.05
keeping informed	2.03
veto over	2.03
party, open-house	8.05
passive-aggressive behavior	7.12
pelvic inflammatory disease	4.14
pentads	2.05, 9.05
period (menstruation)	4.02, 4.04
personal space	9.09
personality, suited to polyamory	1.04
phobias	8.13

Index

phone calls to home	1.08, 3.02, 5.04, 8.08
physical preferences	1.01
PID	4.14
Platinum Rule	6.06
pleasure without penetration	4.12
political activism	8.11

polyamory
    and intentional communities ... 2.07
    and polygamy ... 1.03
    and swinging ... 1.02, 1.07
    bisexuals ... 1.04
    connectedness ... 1.02
    description ... 1.01
    experiment ... 1.06
    extrovert, introvert ... 1.04
    for swingers ... 1.07
    hard work ... 1.01
    homosexuals ... 1.04
    how to suggest ... 6.03, 6.05
    important skills ... 6.01, 6.13
    inexperienced ... 1.06
    introvert, extrovert ... 1.04
    moratoriums ... 1.06, 6.04, 7.13
    not for everyone ... 1.04
    orientation or choice ... 1.04
    personality ... 1.04
    single person ... 2.02
    strength of bond ... 1.04
    suggesting to date ... 6.03
    suggesting to primary ... 6.05
    time limit ... 1.06
    triads and larger ... 2.04
    trial period ... 1.06
    varieties ... 2.01
    when to mention ... 6.03

polyandry ... 1.03
polyfidelity ... 2.04

Index

polygamy	1.03
polygyny	1.03
poly/mono relationships	2.08, 6.07
polyphobia	8.13
polysexuality	6.12
poly-swinger mixed	2.09
powers of attorney	10.03
preferences, physical	1.01
presentations, public	8.12
primary partners meeting secondary	7.08

primary relationship (see also "secondary")
    emotionally dead 3.02
    weak or flawed 3.04

privacy	3.08, 9.09
programming	7.05
projection	1.01, 6.13, 8.13, 10.07
psychotherapy	7.14
PTSD	7.04
pubic lice	4.14
public presentations	8.12
quads	9.04
questionnaire	1.05, App. C
real estate	10.05
reassurance	2.08, 7.07
reinforcement	2.08, 7.07

relationship agreements
    modifying 5.05
    sample agreement 5.06
    sex practices 4.02, 5.04
    sleeping arrangements 5.04
    tacit 7.08
    violations 7.11
    what to cover 5.04
    when to develop 5.02
    who needs 5.01
    written or oral 5.03

Index

relationships
    atomic or molecular 6.06
    barter 6.06, 7.05
    breaking up dyad 7.16
    breaking up secondaries 7.16
    breaking up triad or larger 9.12
    complexity 1.01, 9.02
    couple with couple 2.03
    emotionally dead 2.03
    open or closed 7.08
    primary, maintaining 1.01
    secondary 2.03
religion 8.07
reluctant agreement 7.12
resolving issues 7.01
resources .... 7.01, App. A
risk and benefit balance 4.01
roadblocks to scheduling 7.12
safe sex
    anal 4.06
    dildos and other toys 4.07
    genital 4.04
    more fun 4.12
    oral 4.05
    without penetration 4.12
sandwich approach 7.07
scabies 4.14
scheduling
    general 6.13 6.13, 8.02
    roadblocks to 7.12
schools 8.06
secondaries
    approval by primary 5.04
    being one 2.11
    bringing home 5.04
    dates alone 5.04
    demeaning or pejorative term, considered 2.10

Index

    how much information 5.04
    hypothetical 6.09
    informing 7.08
    introducing to primary 6.09
    maximum number 5.04
    overnight with 5.04
    potential new 3.02
    relevance of term 2.10
    staying overnight 5.04
self-confidence 6.13
self-esteem
    general 6.13
    poor 7.05
separation, effect on children 7.16, 9.12
sex
    anal 4.02, 4.06
    combinations 2.12
    enjoyment 1.02
    genital 4.04
    oral 4.05
    threesomes and moresomes 2.04, 2.12, 6.12
    toys 4.07
sexual hygiene 4.01
sharing .... (see "communication")
single person 2.02
skills 6.13
slander 10.10
sleeping arrangements 5.04
societal norms 5.01
personal space 9.09
speaking
    style 8.12
    to nonpolys 3.10
special friends 8.08
spreading the word 8.11
standing out in crowd 6.13
starting a local group 8.10

364

Index

STDs	4.01, 4.14
stereotypes	8.13
stimulation, digital	5.04
stuck	6.08
subconscious	6.01
subgroups	9.05
support, child	10.06
support groups	7.15

swinging
- changing to poly ... 1.07
- general ... 1.02

syphilis	4.14

talks
- family ... 9.10
- public ... 8.12

Tannen, Deborah	6.02
tattooing	4.01
teamwork	9.03

testing
- DNA, for parentage ... 9.06
- for STDs ... 4.09

therapy	3.04, 7.14
threats, perceived	8.13
threesomes	6.12
toys	4.07
traits	6.13

triads and larger
- bed arrangements ... 9.03
- biological parents ... 9.05, 10.06
- burnout ... 9.01
- catalyst for growth ... 9.01
- children in ... 6.11, 9.03
- complexity ... 1.01, 9.02
- differences from dyads ... 9.02
- discussions ... 9.03
- dynamics ... 2.04, 9.01
- finances ... 9.08

Index

    FMF or MFM 9.03
    leaving 9.12
    living arrangements 9.07
    parental role 9.05
    personal space 9.09
    secondary relationships 2.04
    sexual combinations 9.03
    teamwork 9.03
trial periods 1.06
tribes 2.05, 9.05
trichomoniasis 4.14
trust 6.13
unconscious 6.01
unfaithfulness 7.07
unknown looms 6.09
V 2.04
vaginitis 4.14
varieties 2.01
verification 3.02
veto power 2.03
vibrators 4.07
warts, genital 4.14
waterproof pads 4.04
weak spots 6.01, 6.08, 9.11
what goes around 3.01
wills
    living 10.02
    testamentary 10.04
women, single 1.02
zoning 10.05, 10.08

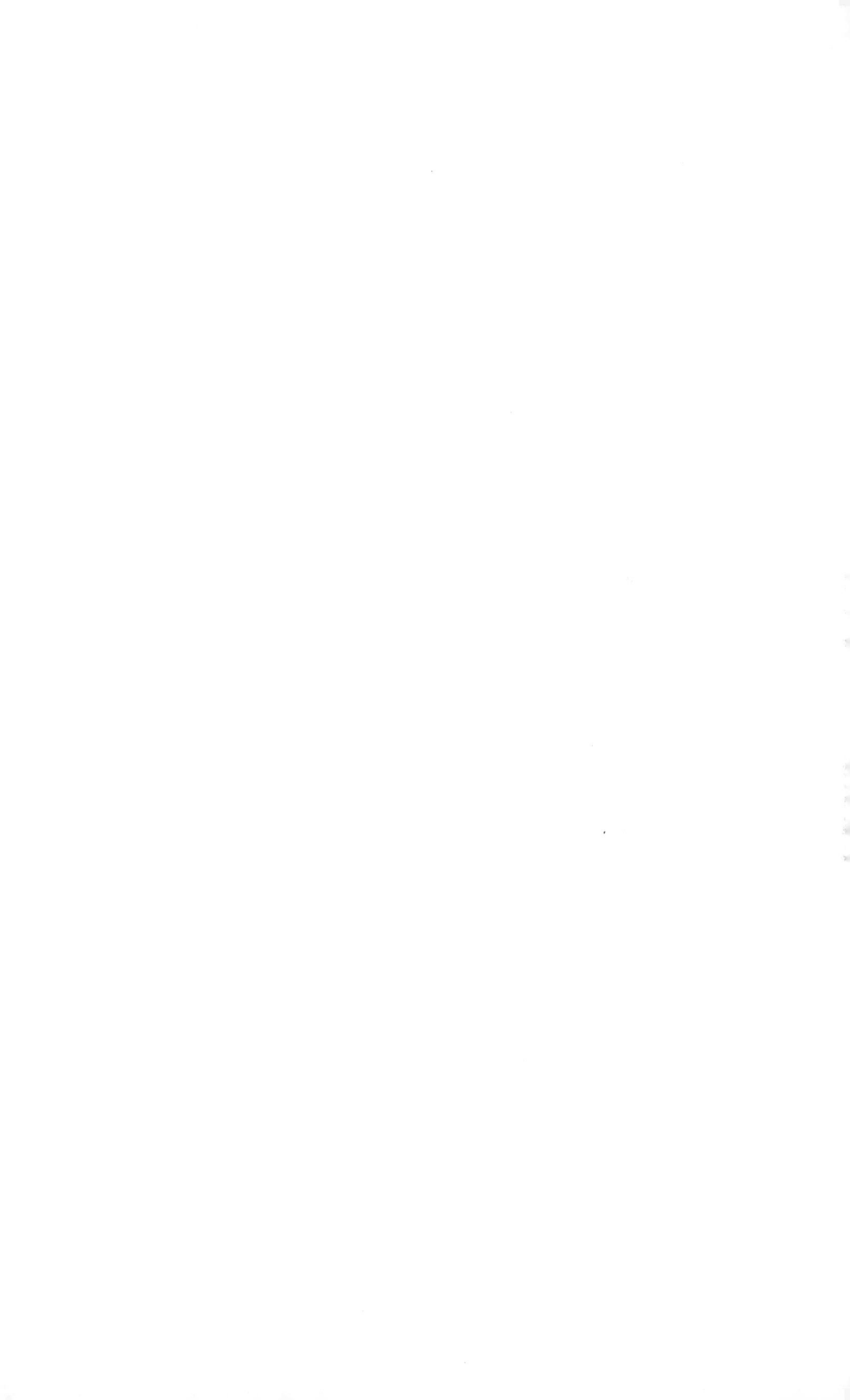